# LIPOEDEMA

*AN EVOLUTIONARY MISMATCH*

**Ahmet Karacalar**



**Illustration**
Victoria Johnson

ISBN: 978-1-949872-81-1

Publisher Cosmo Publishing
UNITED STATES OF AMERICA

May 2023

# LIPOEDEMA

*AN EVOLUTIONARY MISMATCH*

**Biography**

Ahmet Karacalar, Prof.Dr. is specialized in the field of aesthetic, plastic, and reconstructive surgery. He pursued an academic career as the scientific step of his efforts to create an eclectic way of aesthetic surgery. He stayed away from the professorial stereotypes. He makes figurative and abstract bronze sculptures. Amazonizm, Breast, and Aesthetics; The Amazons and the Scream of Matriarchy; Aesthetic Surgery and the Cinderella Tale, Iconoplasty; Lipoedema and Its Treatment are among his other books. He has over fifty international articles, of which he is the first author.

# CONTENTS

*Find your life purpose, if you can't find it,*
*create your life purpose.*

# INTRODUCTION

*Lipoedema is a syndrome that is often mistaken for obesity. This under-recognized health problem is an escalating threat that affects 10 % of the female population in Western countries. Looking at the issue from a more unorthodox perspective, the book mainly focuses on how our evolutionary past contributes to lipoedema, how lipoedema can be explained with the evolution theory's "survival of the fittest," and how we can apply the evolutionary principles to the treatment of lipoedema. Lipoedema certainly needs an unorthodox approach because it is often misdiagnosed, mismanaged, and mistreated. The first lipoedema cases are closely related to the agricultural revolution, which took place in Anatolia, present-day Turkey.*

*I wrote this book during the coronavirus pandemic, but for it, I would not have written it because of my hectic schedule. In March 2019, I operated on a lipoedema patient. She was from a nearby city and was uneventfully discharged from the hospital. Elective operations were forbidden a few days after the surgery, and we got locked down. The patient called me and said she felt dizziness and palpitation. I experienced a profound dilemma between sending her to an emergency department full of covid positive patients or following her with remote patient monitoring at home. I called the fully equipped hospital where the patient underwent surgery in Istanbul. The doctor in the emergency department asked me not to refer the patient because many patients were running high fevers. As someone taking every medical complaint seriously, I was in a confused state of mind. Catching the Covid-19 virus in a patient during recovery would be a catastrophe. Another hospital was found to accept the patient. She needed to be evaluated by the internal medicine doctor, who, unfortunately, was under quarantine. The patient went home because of the fear of catching the virus. After a few stressful days, her vitals became stable. It was a massive relief for me.*

*Lipoedema patients are under a bombardment of information. I often notice this overload causes information anxiety. How do we determine if that information is coming from a credible source? It is obvious to trust literature published in a scientific journal selected for indexing in a trusted database. At the same time, grey literature can be much harder to assess, particularly from commercial sources on websites or blogs.*

*In my culture, it is said that "a madman throws a stone into a well; forty wise men are unable to take it out." Misinformation can be more harmful than we think.*

*The following are basic questions to verify information's reliability and become a conscious internet user. How recent is the information? How recently has the website been updated? Who is the author? What is the publisher's interest in this information? Are there advertisements on the website? Does the author cite references?*

*I added some interesting case reports to this book, which includes my observations and first-hand experiences. Although randomized controlled trials are placed at the top of the hierarchy of evidence-based medicine, case reports have a valuable role in advancing medical knowledge. A single case may provide the basis for more definitive research and is the first link in the chain of evidence. Osler's quote is quite encouraging "Always note and record the unusual…Publish it"*

*In the formal medical training of my generation, the senior professors used to talk about "Sense Clinique." This mesmerizing French-borrowed term, the remnants of Francophile in the latest period of the Ottoman Empire, literally means clinical sense. It was said doctors could diagnose while a patient entered their office. Sens Clinique was a precious gift from a devoted doctor. Unfortunately, it seems to be the reminiscence of the golden age of medicine, which should undoubtedly be revitalized to regain the respectful status of doctors, which has been eroded with the rise of money-driven medicine.*

*The great professors would often remind us of the value of patient-centered care as epitomized in a Hippocratic aphorism "There is no disease, but the patient." Unfortunately, It dies off from the medical profession with the evolution of "modern" medicine dependent on "machines" to diagnose the disease. Let alone taking a good history; even clinical examination is ruled out or skipped to prescribe a wide array of tests. It is undoubtedly not justified even in today's high-speed, high-tech world.*

*Undoubtedly, sophisticated tests are a great asset to modern medicine. These tests are not the necessary use of investigations for a straightforward diagnosis of lipoedema like lymphoscintigraphy or MRI.*

*A doctor should tailor their treatment strategy to the patient's symptoms. This approach is crucial for lipoedema.*

*We should attentively listen to patients to learn their perspectives, remembering that "every patient has a story." There may be much more in a patient's story, including life lessons embedded inside. In my second year of Aegean Medical Faculty, an anatomist used to give us Latin lessons. I clearly remember one of the Latin quotes thought by him. "Bene diagnoscitur, bene curatur." Something that is well diagnosed can be cured well.*

*In the Hellenistic Age, there were two famous schools of medicine- an empirical school at Knidos and a philosophical school of medicine at Cos. A vigorous competition existed between these two schools.*

*Knidos lies at the tip of the Datça peninsula in the southwest corner of western Turkey. The city was an important commercial center and the home of a famous medical school in 700 B.C. It is an extraordinary place that draws me in with its magical energy.*

*The island of Cos is a small Greek island, ten miles from Knidos, opposite the ancient town of Halicarnassus, which is now present day Bodrum in the Aegean region of Turkey. Although it belongs to Greece, it is closer to Turkey than to mainland of Greece. It may be intriguing to note that the two places where two great medical schools were founded and caused plenty of repercussions in medicine, the peninsula of Knidos and the island of Cos, were in the same region.*

*The ancient medical school of Knidos concentrated on the "disease" rather than the patient. In contrast, The Cos school emphasized the "patient" rather than the disease, with great attention to evaluating the physical findings. The chief physician of the medical school of Knidos was Euryphon, who led his school in opposition to the school of Cos.*

*Hippocrates was the master physician of the Cos school and also medicine in general in antiquity. The Cos school had this great doctor who will be referred to as " The Father of Medicine" for his lasting contributions to the field. The Hippocratic School emphasized the clinical doctrines of clinical inspection and observation.*

*Owing to Hippocrates' superiority over Euryphon, the Hippocratic tradition became a part of contemporary medicine, but until recently.*

*Having shifted from Hippocratic medicine and philosophy, today's modern medicine overlooks Hippocrates's aphorism, "There is no disease but the patient." The Cos school of medicine seems to have lost the long-lasting battle, 2500 years later, against the Knidian school of medicine.*

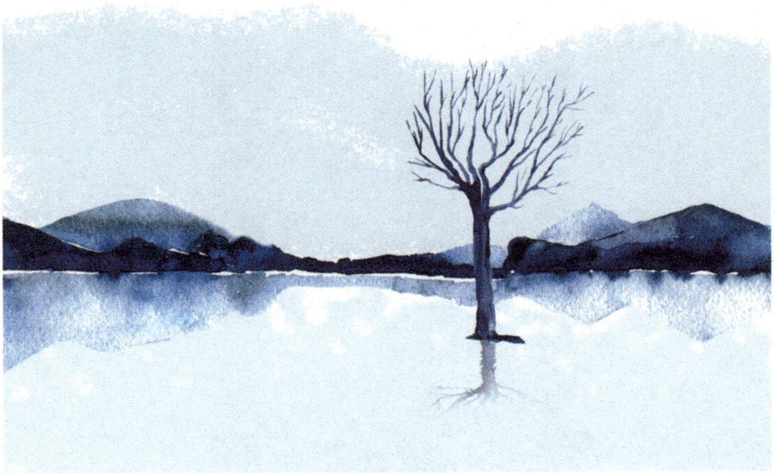

*Figure 1: Survival Instinct*

# PATIENT ZERO: KYBELE

At the Museum of Anatolian Civilizations, Turkey, there is a baked clay of a mother goddess sitting on her throne, flanked by two leopards (Fig. 2). This figurine was unearthed at Çatalhöyük, which UNESCO regarded as the most significant settlement documenting early settled agricultural life. That figurine dating back to 6000 B.C., is regarded as the mother goddess of ancient Anatolia. It symbolizes motherhood, fertility, and abundance. The mother goddess symbol is still well and alive in our culture, woven into the modern Turkish rugs of today.

The figurine of Mother Goddess typically represents a lipoedema patient with diagnostic cuff signs around her ankles, disproportionally accumulated fat in her upper arms and legs, and knees covered with typically lipoedematous fat. The sharp separation between normal and abnormal tissue, a pathognomonic sign in lipoedema, is seen at the ankle and between the hips and waist. Her ptotic breasts and flaccid belly are signs of a recent delivery. The head of the newborn infant between the legs is seen. The Anatolian leopard is a sacred animal and symbolizes her boundless power over nature.

In the Neolithic era, women with lipoedema were certainly respected and sacred figures. The "Survival of the fittest" theory could explain that the women with lipoedema were most successful in surviving and reproducing. Therefore, they were attractive and charming to men. They represented the beauty ideals of the time. Divine power would only survive in famine, giving birth, and breastfeeding. They became Kybele. They were sitting on the throne. They deserved to be worshipped as a fertility goddess.

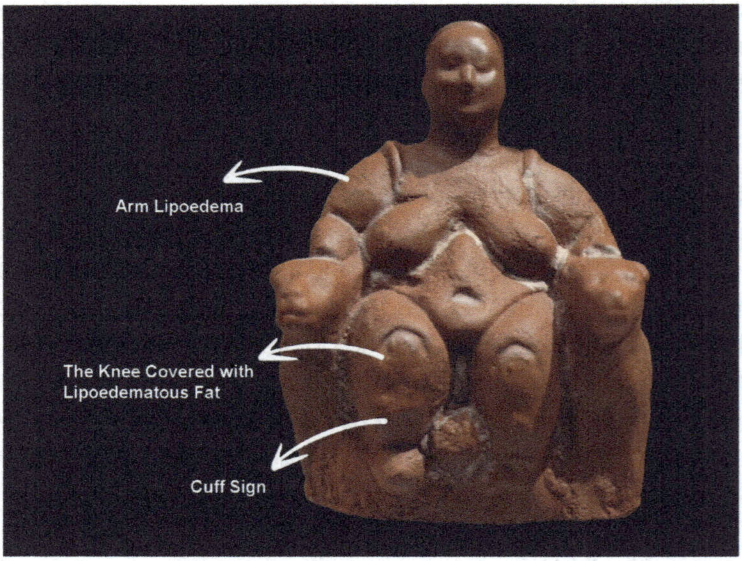


*Figure 2: Kybele*

From an evolutionary perspective, storing fat was once adaptive and enabled us to survive (or sustain fecundity) through periods of famine. Living creatures have different notions of what is attractive. The most colorful feathers in a peacock are taken to guarantee the best way to pass on solid genes to its offspring, and it is a criterium of attractiveness in a peacock.

The surviving traits are not explicitly visible to us. Beauty is the visible version of the surviving traits. Therefore, we have evolved into seeing beauty. Kybele was adopted by the Greeks living in Asia Minor (modern-day Turkey), and she spread from there to mainland Greece, followed by Rome. She protected her holly place until the paradigm shift occurred in beauty norms and was replaced with Artemis, who had today's beauty norms (Fig. 3). Artemis stole the spotlight and became a fertility/childbirth goddess.

"I hypothesize that lipoedema started with the agricultural revolution in Çatalhöyük; it is an evolutionary mismatch."

The region in which the Neolithic farmers started the agricultural revolution is known as Çatalhöyük, the surrounding region of which is still well-known for wheat fields. Before the settlement at Çatalhöyük, humanity had been wanderers for millions of years. Humanity went from a nomadic lifestyle to settled communities in a way that nothing would ever be the same again. It was a significant revolution in history.

Lipoedema developed as part of biological adaptation based on a radically changed lifestyle, a more sedentary life, and changing diet based on kinds of wheat. A sedentary lifestyle must have led to a lower metabolism rate. Because their lifestyle changed from being active all the time (hunting and gathering) to periodic work on the farms and a sedentary lifestyle, they did not need to be as fast, athletic, and muscular as they had. Agriculture and animal husbandry have led to natural human lifestyle changes and shaped modern human genomes (Hehemann et al.). Excess calories combined with a lack of physical activity, a wheat-based, less nutritious diet, and the drastic change in the host–microbiota symbiosis (dysbiosis) in the guts catalyzed lipoedema to manifest. The figurines in the excavations are the archeological supporting evidence of my hypothesis.

We have been farming only for 10,000 years. Comparing human evolution millions of years, we have added grains to our diet in the blink of an eye in evolutionary terms (Figure 4). As we did not adapt to the agricultural revolution, we experienced the industrial revolution. We got hit a double whammy. We have fallen out of sync with our environment with the digital revolution.

Cultural evolution moves faster today than biological evolution, and natural selection cannot correct mismatches. Consequently, we humans suffer from mismatched diseases.

Lipoedema is linked to the agricultural revolution; likewise, obesity is connected to the industrial revolution, which enhanced comfort, reduced movement, and offered easy food availability. Obesity is a disease in modern society. Over the past century, advances in the food industry have directly contributed to the growing worldwide obesity epidemic. Ultra-processed products such as fast food added to the excessive weight gain. Grains and sugar are now readily available in massive quantities year-round, and the consumption of genetically engineered foods has also caused higher rates of obesity.

Ample fat reserves in lipoedematous regions must have sustained nursing and average postnatal growth during seasonal fluctuations in food availability. It is well-known that fat in lipoedema patients is resistant to diet and sports. At the same time, fat in obesity can be burnt off with a calorie-restricted diet. Since the beginning of agriculture, humanity has gone through famine due to drought. In famine, the women with lipoedema must have survived, given birth, and breastfed. Famine imposed selection pressures on the human race. Women require adipose tissue to make up at least 22% of their body weight to keep ovulation and reproduction. When body fat falls below this threshold, estrogen synthesis slows, and fertility is suppressed (Frisch). The genotype of lipoedema must have been evolutionarily successful for women with lipoedema. Those with lipoedematous fat must have better survived times of food scarcity and thus passed on their genes.

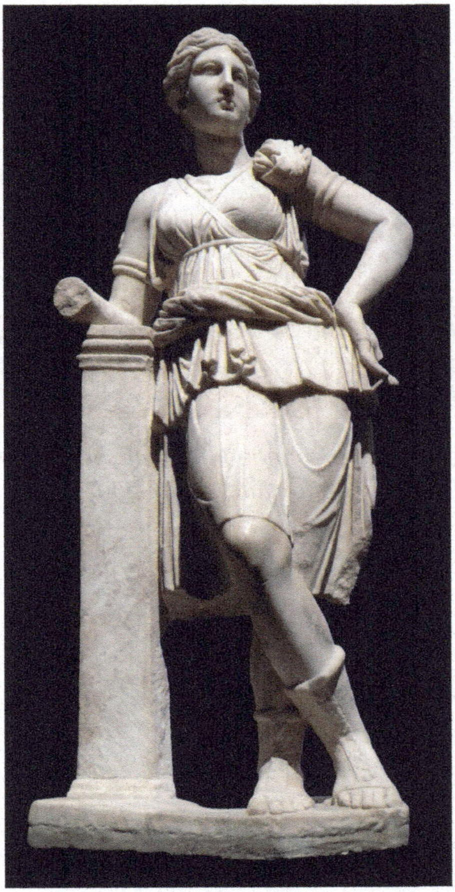

*Figure 3: Artemis, Istanbul Archaeological Museum*

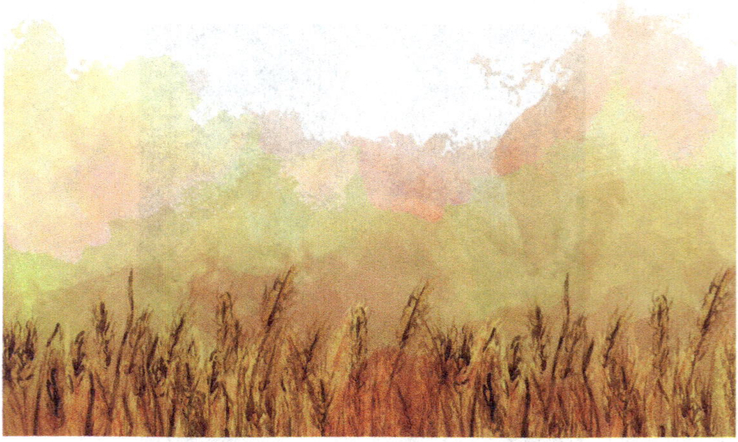

*Figure 4: Wheat changed humanity forever with the agricultural revolution.*

Lipoedema patients are often accused of not sticking to their diets. They are usually in dispute with their husbands or mothers. When I tell them it is resistant to reduction by diet and exercise called persistent fat, I witness how the patients relieve their tensions by nodding to me, "I always keep telling them they are resistant." It is even resistant to bariatric surgery.

Approximately 13 kg fat or 500,000 kJ would theoretically last for 2.4 months. As a result, survival depended not only on fitness, as argued by Darwin, but also on fatness since fatness can guarantee weeks of survival without any food supply. The resistant fat has been an evolutionary benefit to a woman.

In situations with extreme selection pressure, there can be adaptations to diet changes over a short amount of time. Lactose-tolerant people could have better-survived famines like the women with lipoedema. The ability to digest lactose became advantageous to humans. The genetic mutation gave them a significant advantage in nutritional acquisition. They drank the milk of the animals they raised. People with the lactase mutation survive and pass on that gene. The gene encoding an enzyme named lactase shuts down after infancy; when dairy became prevalent, many people evolved a mutation that kept the gene turned on throughout their lives. Owing to this mutation, people adapted themselves to eating dairy by developing lactose tolerance.

Lactose tolerance helped civilizations accelerate human evolution. Ironically Darwin suffered from lactose intolerance without being aware of it. He had vomiting, gut problems, headaches, severe tiredness, skin problems, and depression for over 40 years. It was revealed that all of Darwin's symptoms match systemic lactose intolerance. His family history shows a major inherited component, as with genetically predisposed hypolactasia. Darwin only got better when, by chance, he stopped taking milk and cream. Darwin's illness highlights something else he missed the importance of lactose in mammalian and human evolution (Campbell and Matthews).

According to some scientists, obesity was once adaptive in our evolutionary past. It does not seem to be a plausible hypothesis. Obesity cannot be a biological adaptation of evolution, considering its associated comorbidities. Obesity is a causal factor in numerous severe metabolic and endocrine disorders, including heart disease, diabetes, and some forms of cancer.

In addition, overweight and obese women have higher leptin levels produced in fatty tissue. This has detrimental influences on several human body functions, including reproductive health. In fact, lipoedema was adaptive. The patients with the accumulation of lipoedematous fat around the buttock, hip, and upper thigh must have been at an advantage in evolution. Patients with lipoedema have a lower prevalence of type 2 diabetes and a low risk of dyslipidemia and hypertension. Patients with lipoedema display a less severe cardiovascular profile (De la Torre et al.).

Biologic organisms employ different strategies for metabolic thrift. Torpor, hibernation, reduced metabolic rate, and high rates of caloric intake are a few of the many strategies.

A kind of "thrifty genes" in lipoedema might have helped people to improve energy efficiency. They were passed down from these ancestors of present-day humans.

The agricultural revolution changed the dynamics of society from small clusters of hunter-gatherers to a large community of farmers. The change also brought about an abundance of food, even though seasonal. Crop production led to increases in carbohydrate-rich diets with extensive diet modifications. Decreased variety of food also meant a reduced variety of nutrients in these people's diets. Milk was also added to diets. It caused drastic changes in oral microbiota and gut microbiota. In lipoedema's etiology, microbiota deterioration is blamed on the progress. Some authors reported that the main change in the host–microbiota symbiosis (dysbiosis) likely occurred almost 10,000 years ago, during the Neolithic revolution, also called the "agricultural revolution" (De Filippo et al.; Ottavianiet al.), which might have triggered lipoedema.

Microbiota strongly influences various physiological processes: endocrine and metabolic pathways, immune system regulation, and genome epigenetic changes that affect how your genes work. Gastrointestinal tract–microbiota interactions influence host health by promoting the development and maintenance of the mucosal immune system, protecting against pathogen invasion, and maintaining gastrointestinal tract barrier integrity (Kurashima et al.).

Göbeklitepe, Turkish for "Belly Hill," is rewriting our entire understanding of human history which is located in the Southeastern Anatolia Region of Turkey, lying in Upper Mesopotamia. Göbeklitepe, which dates back around 12,000 years, certainly deserves that description as a milestone in the development of human civilization. This place has the world's oldest temple so far and is regarded as where civilization was born. The social meetings taking place in Göbeklitepe strengthen the idea that people were living just before a significant change in human history, the transition to permanent settlement (Schmidt, 2018).

At Göbeklitepe, the grains look wild, suggesting domestication had not occurred. Gazelle was the primary meat animal. This species was migratory, so a large-scale meat supply was possible in late autumn. The second essential species were aurochs.

The impressive T-shaped pillars are the characteristic element of Göbeklitepe´s architecture (Figure 5). They are clearly an abstract interpretation of the human body. Most sculptures are intended to be enjoyed from various viewpoints. Therefore, we should walk around a statue to fully comprehend it. From a distance, the T pillars seem to be abstract sculptures. But, from a closer angle, the pillars are stylized depictions of people, physically fit figures with no trace of lipoedema.

The primary purpose of stylization is to make the art motif more comprehensible to the viewer. The stylization method in art requires separating from the image all the surplus interfering with clear visual perception. It aims to draw attention to their previously hidden aesthetic or nature and evoke corresponding emotional intensity.

Fashion illustration is one of the striking examples of a stylized perspective. When sketching their ideas, designers elongate the model's height. They distort their body proportions, such as narrow waist and long limbs, in order to create an artistic effect or reveal the essence of the depicted objects.

I applied this method to one of my sculptures, which is closely relevant to the book. As you see in Figure 6, I made an exaggerated form of the breasts as one of the striking symbols of fertility, implying that it had undergone a silicon implant surgery. Her body was incongruous with her giant, well-shaped breasts. I called it a modern goddess. Despite her thin body, she can still be fertile owing to the level modern medicine has reached.

About two thousand years later, in a region called Çatalhöyük, situated seven hundred kilometers north of Göbekli Tepe, the agricultural revolution took place. Were they the descendants of local hunter-gatherers who adopted the farming way of life?

Çatalhöyük is known in archaeology as a proto-city, a link between the cave-dwellings of prehistoric hunter-gatherers and the early urban constructions. Çatalhöyük was constructed with the house complexes. The inhabitants of Çatalhöyük walked around on the settlement's rooftops and climbed into houses with ovens.

There were no streets or passageways. They climbed into houses with ovens on their southern side to let out the smoke and take in the sunlight and fresh air. All houses were similar in size, and none of them looked significantly larger. Çatalhöyük features an egalitarian model of society in many respects. No kings or leaders or groups of elites have been identified yet.

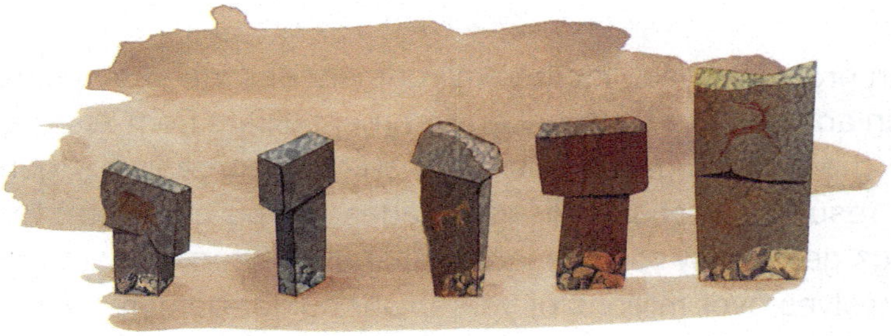

*Figure 5: T-shaped pillars, Göbeklitepe*

In Çatalhöyük, the people domesticated wheat. How do we know this? The DNA analysis of charred wheat grains from Çatalhöyük and the comparison of these wheat grains with contemporary wheat species showed that the Çatalhöyük wheat stock contained hexaploid wheat, which is similar to contemporary hexaploid wheat species.

The hunting-gathering communities in Europe were replaced entirely with Anatolian farmers. Migrants spread north and west, bringing their specialist farming skills and the genetic inheritance of lipoedema. Archaeogenetic research has demonstrated that European Neolithic farmers were descended primarily from Anatolian Neolithic farmers (Lazaridis et al.).

An organism best fits the environment described by its genes. When an organism's current environment differs from its ancestral one, the environment's mismatch with the organism's genome may result in functional disadvantages for the organism. Human beings' genetically conditioned nutritional requirements established themselves over millions of years. Our hunter-gatherer ancestors ate a diet markedly different from that of agriculturally dependent contemporary human beings (Sebastian et al.).

Humans gradually evolved over 6 million years as "hunter-gatherers" and developed symbiotic relationships with nature, breathed fresh air, drank fresh water, and ate fresh foods. Anatomically, we remain broadly "paleolithic."

In 1814, Ivan Krylov, "the Russian La Fontaine," a Russian poet and writer, wrote a fable entitled "The Inquisitive Man." After the voluminous discussion above, I want to share a paragraph from the book which will have a calming effect on your mind.

*Good day, dear friend; where do you come from?*

*"From the Museum, where I have spent three hours, I saw everything they have there and examined it carefully. So much*

*have I seen to astonish me that, if you believe me, I am neither strong enough nor clever enough to describe it fully? Upon my word, it is the palace of wonders. How rich Nature is an invention! What birds and beasts haven't I seen there! What flies; butterflies, cockroaches, little bits of beetles! -some like emeralds, others like coral. And what tiny cochineal insects, others like coral. And what tiny cochineal insects! Why some of them are smaller than a pin's head?"*

*"But did you see the elephant? What did you think it looked like? I'll be bound; you felt like you were looking at a mountain."*

*"Are you quite sure it's there?" "Quite sure."*

*"Well, brother, you mustn't be too hard upon me, but to tell the truth, I didn't remark the elephant.*

*The tale tells the story of a man who visits a museum. Although he can see all the peculiarities and details of the most miniature objects on display, he completely misses the presence of an elephant.*

We fail to notice the big picture in lipoedema. My hypothesis helps fall things in place.

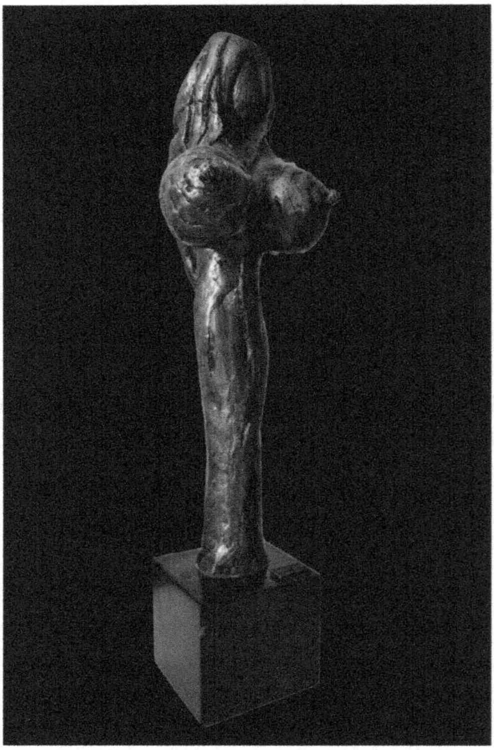

*Figure 6: Modern Goddess*

# LIPOEDEMA: WHAT REALLY IS IT?

Lipoedema is a disease with high prevalence but low recognition. Likely, the condition is often misdiagnosed or wrongly diagnosed as lifestyle-induced obesity or lymphedema. Putting it mildly, lipoedema is generally unknown to medical providers. I even heard from my patients there were doctors saying, "There is no such a disease." The literature has presented inconsistent data regarding the prevalence of lipoedema. However, lipoedema is believed to affect nearly 11% of adult women.

I pointed out the evolutionary basis of lipoedema in the above sentences, which will improve the understanding of the disease in its treatment and management and provide new insights into it. Evolutionary principles can be employed in tackling public health issues, such as using hormone replacement therapy in postmenopausal women. Its association with increased breast cancer risk can be explained by the marked difference between modern-day reproductive patterns, and hence hormone exposure throughout life, and that which occurred in our evolutionary past.

Descartes, the originator of Cartesian doubt, put all beliefs, ideas, thoughts, and matter in doubt and said, "If you would be a real seeker after truth, it is necessary that at least once in your life you doubt, as far as possible, all things."

Dogmatism is everywhere, even in science and medicine. The dominant beliefs can monopolize scientific studies and prevent the truth from revealing.

There is much confusion about the description of lipoedema. Let's discuss it from the perspective of Cartesian skepticism. In an effort to analyze etymologically, the word lipoedema can break down into two parts: lipo and edema. The word lipo derives from the Greek lipos, meaning fat. Oedema means swelling caused by an accumulation of fluid. Oedema is sometimes spelled as edema. This generic name does not reflect its pathophysiological reality.

The word lupus is a misnomer for lupus disease, which is a chronic inflammatory autoimmune disease. Lupus means wolf in Latin, and it referred to lupus disease caused by cutaneous tuberculosis before the 19th century that was thought to resemble the bites of a wolf.

Columbus made landfall in the continent of America, considering that he had reached India. Therefore, he dubbed the native people Indians. This misnomer still refers to indigenous peoples throughout the Americas. Native Americans were largely hunters and gatherers, even in some domestication cases. They were typical of hunter-gatherers, physically fit and healthy.

Columbus wrote in his diary. "They were very well built, with very handsome bodies and very good faces," "They do not carry arms or do not know them...They should be good servants."

Owing to brutalism and infectious diseases, most of the hunter-gatherer population was decimated within decades.

The Native American diet before European contact was relatively nutrient-dense, incorporating varied macro-nutrients and micro-nutrients through hunting and gathering practices and indigenous forms of horticulture that were subsequently disrupted (Armelagos et al.).

In the centuries after European contact, many Native American communities were forced to move away from their paleo diets. The decline in Native American health and fertility coincides with European colonization.

In lipoedema, the lipoedemic fat accumulates symmetrical, mainly in the extremities from the hips and shoulders down.

However, the adipose tissue is not the only diseased tissue in lipoedema. Adipose tissue is condemned because the loose connective tissue is composed of roughly only 80% fat. Some women with lipoedema also have higher aortic distensibility and strain, reliable characteristics of arterial elasticity, and are also suggestive of connective tissue changes consistent with hypermobility.

The whole thing related to the pathogenesis of lipoedema points to the interstium, although the debate is continuing whether it is a new organ or not. The interstitium is a contiguous fluid-filled space existing between a structural barrier, such as a cell wall or the skin, and internal structures, such as organs, including muscles and the circulatory system.

The interstitium not only represents a passive conduit system for the flux of fluid and solutes but also functions as a highly dynamic and complex structure. The interstitial space is the primary source of lymph and is a significant fluid compartment in the body.

Experts have long thought parts of the body (like skin, veins, and arteries, and the lining around muscles) contain collagen walls, the main component of connective tissue. Instead, as the new study points out, those "walls" are not walls at all. Instead, they're spaces filled with fluid that are simply supported by collagen. Those spaces are the interstitium.

In a new study, researchers claim that the interstitium — fluid-filled spaces in tissue that are connected throughout the body — should be considered a new "organ" and that these spaces may play a major part in what goes on in your body.

The interstitium, which is found all over our bodies, from the skin to muscles to our digestive system, was underrated, and its function was oversimplified, saying it acts as a kind of shock absorber or a passive conduit system for the flux of fluid and solutes, about one-sixth of the total volume of the body in the interstitium.

It turned out that the interstitium was a crucial structure. Researchers did not notice it because the way they obtained tissue samples seemed to have destroyed a crucial part of the tissue. The fluid-filled pockets would leak and collapse when removed and preserved, obscuring all evidence of the interstitium.

This reminds me of Erasistratus' anatomic dissection. He believed the arteries were full of air and carried the spirit. Two hundred years later, famed physician Galen, who treated gladiators returning from their fights, demonstrated that arteries contained blood, not air. Once the heart stops, the blood in the arteries drains away, filled with air. Almost everything that was once a total mystery is common knowledge today.

Capillary filtration drives fluid flow into the interstitium, which not only assists the transport of nutrients through tissues but also plays important roles in tissue morphogenesis and remodeling, regulation of vascular function, formation of new lymph vessels, tumor biology, and immune cell trafficking.

Conditions characterized by abnormally low interstitial fluid flow may also induce dramatic changes in cell function. This results in excessive fluid accumulation in the extravascular compartment in the absence of standard interstitial convection patterns and pathologic changes that cause chronic swelling of the interstitial compartment and precipitate inflammation and fibrosis, adipocyte growth, and lipid accumulation. Excessive accumulation of interstitial fluid may compromise cellular metabolism in the swollen tissue. Edema formation also limits the diffusional removal of potentially toxic by-products of cellular metabolism.

In a James Cameron movie, Alita, Christoph Waltz plays Doctor Dyson Ido, the cybersurgeon. Actually, his character was the prototype of a futuristic plastic surgeon. He was fixing and transplanting cybernetic parts for patients. It sounds too far-fetched. Would you believe a surgeon in New York operating on a patient in France with robotic tools and wireless networking instead of human hands? Two telesurgeons in New York City successfully removed a patient's gallbladder 6,000 kilometers away in France in 2001.

New job specialties emerge while old careers die off because of changing technology and innovations. The same dynamic applies to medicine. My futuristic prediction is that the interstitium specialists will be among the new specialties or sub-specialties in the not-too-far future.

Based on the arguments above, it is reasonable to conclude that lipoedema, as an evolutionary mismatch, is a chronic, progressive, hereditary syndrome of the interstitium in extremities.

Since it is obvious that the word lipoedema is a misnomer, how would we call it? I would say "Inflammatory interstitial syndrome."

# IS LIPOEDEMA A HEREDITARY CONDITION?

Lipoedema is almost certainly a hereditary condition because of its positive family history. % 64 prevalence is the highest for a family history of lipoedema. When I ask patients if there is anybody with similar symptoms in their families, they sometimes say they are the only lipoedema patient among their relatives. Still, when I examine the other members of the family, I always make the diagnosis of lipoedema in various stages.

They respond negatively because they are in their earlier stages and don't accept their condition as a disease. Is Lipoedema hereditary or genetic? Until now, you may have assumed that these two words are interchangeable. Genetic diseases may or may not be hereditary. Hereditary diseases are passed on from one generation to another through defective genes. However, there are occasions when a trait or feature is genetic and not hereditary.

# IS LIPOEDEMA PAINFUL?

I sometimes examine stage 2 patients with no pain, who complain about just tension feeling due to swelling, although they present the fundamental characteristics of the disease. Aren't they lipoedema? or a different entity of disease? Herbst et al. reported four patients with lipoedema denied having any pain. The painful clinical picture of lipoedema might be preceded by a pain-free stage.

The syndrome appears to be linked to abnormalities in the interaction between certain glands – the hypothalamus, pituitary, and adrenal glands – and the nervous system, known as a type of stress axis. The abnormalities in this stress axis, which controls our reactions to stress, injury, and trauma, may explain why certain people experience pain differently.

Pressure pain is caused by the accumulation of water in the fat cells. The increase in volume exerts pressure on the surrounding tissue and creates tension. Consequently, the skin reacts painfully to contact and pressure. The further lipoedema progresses, the stronger the symptoms can become. Legs, arms, or hips can also hurt without pressure as the circumference increases.

A dropping row of dominoes is sometimes used to explain a series of symptoms as an analogy in medicine. If you give the first one a nudge in the domino line, the next domino in the line is knocked over, and the immediate preceding domino causes the fall of each domino. The reaction continues until all collapse. Diabetes is a prime example of this domino effect. The harm extends to any organ when it is not well handled. The cumulative effect created when one event sets off a chain of similar events is a domino effect on health. How to Set the Dominos Back Up before an irreversible stage? This topic is the matter of another chapter.

Unlike acute pain, this condition does not disappear after your initial injury or illness has healed. Sometimes pain evolves into a poorly understood condition known as chronic pain syndrome. It's marked by pain that lasts longer than six months and is often accompanied by anger and depression, anxiety, loss of sexual desire, low back pain, headaches, joint pain, muscle ache, and burning or tingling pain in different parts of the body.

Lipoedema is also a chronic disease. The following are some of the symptoms of stress that you may experience with chronic illness, body aches, fatigue, disturbed sleep, sadness, irritability, anxiety, and headaches. It is obvious that these are also overlapping with the lipoedema symptoms.

Most lipoedema patients have these symptoms, which are attributed to the disease. It may be the symptoms of lipoedema, chronic pain syndrome, chronic illness syndrome, or a mixture of them.

Lipoedema is a chronic disease. Chronic diseases are defined broadly as conditions that last more than one year.

# CONFUSION IN LIPOEDEMA STAGES

Lipoedema is classified mainly into four clinical stages based on morphological appearance. Stage 1: a smooth skin surface with homogenous thickening of the subcutis; Stage 2: a bumpy, wave-like skin surface with nodular structures in the thickened subcutis; Stage 3: an increase in nodular changes and overhanging masses of tissue. Stage 4 is characterized by the development of lymphedema. In my opinion, it is a problematic classification. The texture always is not always in accordance with the severity of the disease. I sometimes observe that even a stage 1 patient may suffer from disturbing pain. This classification does not also take the diameter or tissue thickness into consideration. A patient in stage 1 may have a thicker leg than a stage 2 patient. I remember some patients in stage 1, where fat aspiration was challenging due to fibrosis.

It was a bitter experience for me to learn what fibrotic lipoedema was. It was a long time ago. I operated on a lipoedema patient who was stage 2. On the examination, her skin was tight, similar to lipoedema patients with muscular hypertrophy who exercised too much to burn off the fat. The pinchable tissue was about 10 cm in the calf and was worth the liposuction. During the operation, the tip of the cannula felt stone-hard fibrotic tissue. I experienced similar situations, particularly in the cases who tried very strict diets. The tissue was like a dried fruit that had lost its water. Fibrotic lipoedema is a new entity deserving a different approach, although fibrosis is present in all stages of lipoedema. Lymphostatic fibrosis begins as a high protein accumulation of swelling that gradually attracts fat cells, which promotes the conversion of liquid edema into fatty tissue. Further accumulation of fluid in the setting of decreased oxygen tension leads to fibrosis.

Fibrosis forms around the subcutaneous fat cells, creating nodules. These can range in size from a grain of rice to the size of walnuts or even larger. If lipoedema progresses, the nodules can adhere to each other, creating large, lumpy, painful masses. In the later stages of lipoedema, large pendulous lobules can form, making it challenging to find well-fitting clothing and interfering with sitting, standing, or walking.

Some lipoedema patients have joint hypermobility (especially of the knee), which ultimately causes joint damage. Loss of skin elasticity and temperature in the affected area usually coexist. Some patients have gastrocnemius muscle hypertrophy. The treatment and symptoms of the patient with very loose and tight tissue are quite different. This classification system does not address these issues.

# IS LIPOHYPERTOPHY A PRECURSOR TO LIPOEDEMA?

Teenage patients usually have lipohypertrophy, which may be a precursor to lipoedema. Their mothers often say, “We had the same legs as our daughters, which turned to lipoedema. Lipohypertrophy can develop into lipoedema; however, the exact triggers of disease transition are unknown. Lipohypertrophy differs from lipoedema stage 1 with no existing symptoms. Disease progression is not predictable and, therefore, may vary case-to-case basis. A homogenous increase in subcutaneous fatty tissue and the skin is still smooth. Because lipohypertrophy has no symptoms, it is easily dismissed.

The lipoedema patients sometimes ask me how they can protect their children against lipoedema since they carry the same genetic inheritance. I recommend that they prevent their children from the gain weight. Weight loss reduces the volume of fat cells but not their number. During childhood and adolescence, the number of fat cells can increase or decrease, but after the teen years, the body aims at keeping the number of fat cells constant. If you are obese as a teenager or young adult, when the body settles on its preferred fat cell number, it is likely to result in a greater number of fat cells in adulthood and a potential life-long weight struggle. We have a fixed number of fat cells as an adult. New fat cells are constantly created and destroyed, but the body maintains a fixed number set during adolescence. Therefore, it is so crucial to prevent childhood obesity.

The greater number of fat cells in formerly obese people may be a factor in their tendency to regain the weight they lost. The exact amount of fat is distributed across a larger number of fat cells versus a small number of fat cells with the same weight and volume.

# EVERY PATIENT HAS A STORY

“Listen to your patient; he is telling you the diagnosis.” This was what Osler taught his students in the late 19th century. Despite the considerable advances in medicine, this axiom still holds as true.

Narrative medicine uses a patient-centered approach to understand the meaning of the patient’s reasoning. For instance, doctors and patients can use the word cellulite, but that does not signify that both share the same meaning. Narrative medicine finds its best application in lipoedema, while time constraints for a surgeon are a barrier to improved communication.

“Beneath the Wheel” by Herman Hesse points out the lost childhood to the scholastic education system. It hints that we live up to our parent’s expectations. It also gives a good example of patient-centered care, epitomized in the Hippocratic aphorism: “There is no disease but the patient.”

The book is about an ambitious boy who slowly breaks down and crushes beneath the wheel of the rigid education system when facing the pressure of the adult world.

Hans would go swimming in the lake, play with his bunnies, interact with his friends, celebrate fairs, take a nice walk through the forest, or spend the day with his favorite activity: fishing.

For three years, his teachers, the vicar, his father, and the headmaster urged him unceasingly, allowing him no rest. He loses his friends; the bunnies are eaten, and fishing is no longer allowed or any other activity.

Hans gets a burn-out in boarding school in an atmosphere of constant tension, pressure, and vast social differences. He suffers from severe headaches accompanied by other symptoms, including change in temperament, lack of appetite, nightmares or difficulty sleeping, temporary motor weakness, concentration problems, dizziness, and suicidal thoughts.

A district physician tends to underestimate his difficulties as a "slight nervous disorder, due principally to his growing" or a "passing condition–light dizzy spells," ignoring Hans's personal life beyond his medical conditions, thus ushering in the tragic end of the novel.

The doctor should encourage the patient to express her story adequately and in her own words without controlling or interfering. Conversation with a lipoedema patient necessitates active listening.

# DIAGNOSIS IN LIPOEDEMA

An experienced doctor can diagnose a patient with the naked eye (visual diagnosis) since lipoedema is characterized by a characteristic stature. The extremities (arms and legs) are usually more voluminous and do not harmonize with a slender upper body, a narrow waist, and delicate wrists and ankles.

It consists of a set of objective and subjective symptoms and signs correlated with each other.

- Tenderness
- Varicose veins
- Knee pain
- Edema
- Numbness
- Skin changes
- Pain
- Fatigue
- Brain fog or difficulty with cognition
- Hypermobility
- Gait abnormalities and leg joint issues
- Psychosocial distress
- Susceptibility to bruising
- Cold foot
- Hot or burning sensation
- Valgus deformities of the feet
- Flat feet
- Comorbidities like obesity, hypothyroidism, migraine, and depression.

The tissue tenderness characteristic of lipoedema can be checked with the pinch test, which often feels very unpleasant in the affected areas but causes no pain elsewhere.

Specific lipoedema diagnostic tests are not available. Diagnosis is thus dependent on examination and history. Therefore, at times, it may not only cause the patient to lose precious moments but may also incur a lot of unnecessary needless costs.

The first manifestation of lipoedema may be the filling of the retro-malleolar sulcus on both lower extremities.

Characteristics are bilateral symmetrical fat deposition confined to the legs, thighs, and buttocks, with sparing of the feet, which results in a “reverse shouldering” effect, also known as the “cuff sign.”

A well-known test pinching the skin over the dorsum of the second toe base (Stemmer sign) is a helpful diagnostic technique to differentiate lipoedema from lymphedema; thickened skin that is difficult to raise off the underlying tissue is considered diagnostic for lymphedema.

It may be helpful to confirm the diagnosis by MRI or high-resolution cutaneous ultrasonography. MRI images usually display diffuse fatty hypertrophy around the bilateral lower extremities without skin abnormalities in patients with lipoedema.

# MENDEL'S BEANS AND LIPOEDEMA

The texture of lipoedematous tissue is described as the nodular "beans in a bag" feel of the fat in lipoedema. Ironically, we can better understand lipoedema's genetic origin if we discuss Mendel's beans (Figure 7).

In computers, information is stored using 0 and 1 as their alphabet. In humans, A-G-C-T letters are the codes. Data is stored in DNA as a code using four different kinds of molecules. Adenine (A), guanine (G), cytosine (C), and thymine (T). A gene is a short section of DNA.

Imagine that you have a collection of cookbooks on your bookshelves. Each recipe in the cookbooks is like a gene. The chromosomes, continuing this analogy, are like bookshelves.

Genes are found on tiny spaghetti-like chromosomes. Chromosomes are found inside the cells. Matryoshka nesting dolls provide a good analogy for these structures. The outermost doll represents the cell, the others nucleus-chromosomes-genes-DNA sequentially.

Your genes are the instruction manual that tells cells how to function your cells and makes your body work properly. Every human has around 20,000 genes that carry the information that determines your traits.

Mendel, known as the "father of modern genetics," discovered the basic principles of heredity through experiments in his monastery's garden. Mendel crossed varieties of peas that differed in one trait. He found that the inheritance was not blending, and all plants were tall. In Mendel's terms, one character was dominant. and the other recessive. Furthermore, when the hybrid plants were crossed, the recessive character reappeared.

Because lipoedema genetic inheritance is based on more than one gene, it is non-Mendelian. Lipoedema does not follow strict rules of inheritance. It means they are not solidly based on inherited genes; even it can skip a generation. Polygenic Genetic disorders are associated with the effects of multiple genes in combination with lifestyles and environmental factors. Environmental factors regulate the human genome by activating and deactivating genes. It is described as "If the genome is the light bulb, environmental factors are "like a dimmer switch rather than a light switch," (Dr. Spector's analogy). On a pedigree, polygenic diseases tend to "run in families," they are not compatible with Mendelian theory. These explanations perfectly fit lipoedema. There needs to be a trigger to activate these genes. If the genes are not activated, the body does not respond by allowing the disease process to occur. Recently Szél, et al. proposed a lipoedema theory in which lipoedema is an estrogen-regulated polygenetic disease, manifesting in parallel with feminine hormonal changes and leading to vasculopathy and lymphangiopathy. These defective genes are suspected of causing primary endothelial barrier dysfunction and lymphangiopathy.

In lipoedema, another affected immediate family member has been reported in up to 60% of women. This is compatible with an autosomal dominant inheritance with incomplete penetrance in which an affected parent has a 50% chance of passing lipoedema to their child. An autosomal dominant disorder occurs when only one defective copy of an autosomal gene is required to cause disease. A person with an autosomal dominant disorder has a 50% chance of having an affected child with one mutated gene in one of the parents.

We can draw a parallelism between lipoedema and obesity in terms of their genetic background. The genetic contribution to obesity is well established. Common obesity is polygenic, involving complex gene-gene and gene-environment interactions.

More studies are required to determine lipoedema's genetic basis accurately. No genetic tests for molecular diagnosis of lipoedema are currently available. We will discuss genetic counseling in lipoedema in the near future to prevent disease progression in children of lipoedema patients.

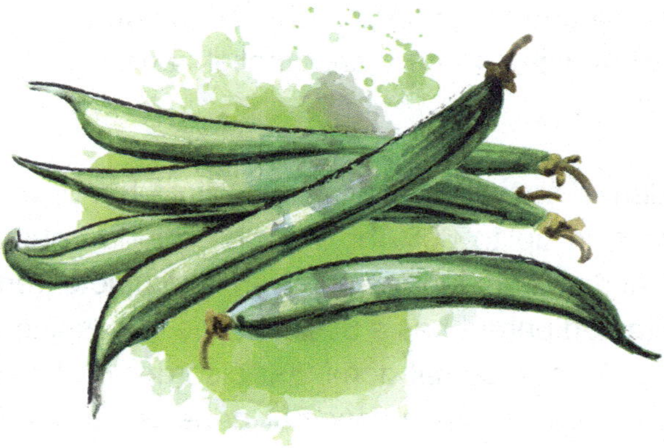

*Figure 7: Lipoedema does not follow strict rules of inheritance.*

# PATHOGENES

You may ask why understanding the disease is needed for the patients who are the primary reader of this book. It is clear that understanding the pathophysiology of the disease is important for healthcare providers of lipoedema to develop new treatment strategies.

However, a conscious patient might be a teacher of a doctor. In our culture, a proverb that says, "Don't ask the doctor; ask the having experienced." The patient who is knowledgeable about lipoedema will also teach other patients or share valuable observations with her doctor. In the 1950s, the mistake of a patient led to an important scientific discovery in Siberia. You probably saw the external fixator devices consisting of still rings, rods, and wires that immobilize bones to allow a fracture to heal properly. The patients are instructed to adjust the fixator several times a day by turning small knobs. Dr. Ilizarov started his career treating some patients in Siberia who had suffered fractures from the Second World War. He designed an external fixator and successfully treated his first patient with a tibial non-union, effectively treating non-unions of bones with compression. His outstanding results significantly reduced healing time. One of his patients lengthened his frame rather than compressing it because the nuts on the frame were accidentally turned in the opposite direction. A non-union, which was supposed to be treated by compression osteogenesis (pushing together bone segments to try and stimulate new bone growth), was given the opposite treatment, pulling the bone apart instead of pushing it together. Dr. Ilizarov observed the new bone formation and discovered distraction osteogenesis, the ability of bone to regenerate by distraction (pulling apart). This patient's mistake became the mainstay of all newly developing treatment methods for a wide variety of conditions.In lipoedema, the loose connective tissue is the diseased part. 'Where is it found in the body?' and 'What is a normal loose connective tissue?'

To understand lipoedema, it is necessary to understand the loose connective tissue. You also need to familiarize yourselves with the terms involved in the lymphatic system and inflammatory processes.

As an analogy, we can draw a parallel between loose connective tissue and the minestrone soup. Like vegetables embedded in a thick soup, loose areolar tissue has cells and a viscous matrix embedded in it. Loose connective tissue includes areolar, reticular, adipose tissues, collagen fibers, elastic fibers, and reticular fibers.

Fibroblasts, adipocytes, and mesenchymal cells are fixed cells that remain permanently within the connective tissue. Other cells move in and out of the connective tissue in response to chemical signals.

# SPONGE OF OUR SKIN: GROUND SUBSTANCE

It forms a matrix like a sponge that absorbs lots of water, and they are good at resisting compressive forces. The ground substance consists mainly of water, whose major role is to provide a communication and transport route (by diffusion) between tissues. Ground substance is made of polysaccharides, specifically hyaluronic acid, which attracts and traps available moisture forming the clear, viscous, and colorless matrix.

COLLAGEN

Collagen fibers, while flexible, give resilience and strength to the tissue. These fibers hold connective tissues together, even during the body's movement. Like a suspension bridge cable, collagen imparts toughness and strength to connective tissue. It is collagen that helps keep your skin from tearing apart when someone pinches you. In some lipoedema patients, the skin is quite loose. They try everything to tighten their skins. From my observations, I can say that the skin of lipoedema patients smoking cigarettes, giving birth, following a vegan diet, and over 40 is looser and softer. It is no surprise smokers have loose skin since the chemicals in tobacco destroy collagen and elastin. Our body naturally produces less collagen as we age, which can contribute to dry skin, wrinkles, and less skin elasticity. Vegans usually have loose skin due to a lack of animal proteins in their diet.

# RUBBER BANDS OF OUR SKIN: ELASTIN

Elastin provides softness and elasticity to the skin, forming a three-dimensional network between the collagen fibers. It is responsible for allowing tissues in the body to "snap back" to their original shape after being stretched or contracted. For this reason, it is often compared to a rubber band. The main property of elastin is that it will return to its original shape after being stretched or compressed. Elastin fibers lose their resilience, and the skin does not snap back as well, resulting in the sagging we see around the eyes, jawline, and neck.

Elastin is found in artery walls and, of course, in the skin. Imagine how blood vessels expand, for instance, when the blood pumps through but then contracts again as when the blood leaves the vessels.

We often hear about these two proteins in skin care because they work together to give skin its shape and firmness.

Elastosis, as a form of degenerative disease, is mainly caused by prolonged and excessive sun exposure. In this condition, abnormal elastin accumulates in the dermis of the skin. It changes the skin's strength and elasticity. Women who are overexposed to the sun because of tan skin obsession do not age gracefully.

Lipoedema symptoms get worse among women who smoke. The nicotine in cigarettes impairs blood flow to your skin by narrowing the blood vessels. The skin does not get as much oxygen and nutrients as it requires. Chemicals in tobacco also damage collagen and elastin, which are fibers that give your skin its strength and elasticity, leading to skin beginning to sag prematurely.

Too much sugar intake converts the collagen into an unstable type 1, which is more vulnerable and can be easily broken down, thus can lead to premature aging.

# INFLAMMATION: UNNOTICED FIRE WITHIN US

Inflammation is a double-edged sword. It is a defense mechanism of the body. Without it, wounds would never heal, and microbes would win the war. Where the body is injured or infected, inflammation starts with plasma and white blood cells. You can feel the signs of such inflammations with five cardinal signs: redness, heat, swelling, pain, and loss of function. Chronic, low-grade, or age-related inflammation is not the kind you can feel.

Obesity and its complications, including high cholesterol, type 2 diabetes, coronary heart disease, high blood pressure, and stroke, have been shown to be associated with chronic inflammation. Lipoedema is also an inflammatory adipocyte growth (hypertrophy), especially if accompanied by vascular supply insufficiency, which leads to adipocytes hypoxia and, consequently, the production of reactive oxygen species; this may cause oxidative stress, damaging cell structures and triggering an inflammatory response. Another side effect of the inflammation is that the transformation of T4 into T3 is diminished. T3 is the metabolically active hormone; its decrease might cause a limited triglyceride release, building up more and more lipids inside the adipocyte.

Discoloration may refer to inflammation of the dermis with melanin accumulation within the dermis. It appears to affect darker-skinned patients with greater frequency and severity. Another theory is hemosiderin triggered by extravasation of the deposition of red cells escaping from the vessels. Another reason for discoloration is livedo reticularis which points to a reticular discoloration of the skin that is reddish-violet and primarily affects the limbs. It is caused by interrupted blood flow in the dermal arteries, either due to spasms, inflammation, or vascular obstruction.

# CAPILLARY MICROCIRCULATION

Macrocirculation is well-known, but most people are unaware of microcirculation. Capillary microcirculation is damaged in lipoedema. What is microcirculation? How can we repair it?

I am sure most of us once splashed, sprayed, and soaked the other kids with the garden hose. When we were little, this could not be done by simply holding the hose out toward them because the water would only run out of the end and onto the ground. We all had to use our thumbs to block a portion of the hose's opening to make the water come out faster. The water spray is increased when the hose opening is blocked because the fluid increases speed when it flows through a narrower space. The same thing happens in rivers as they change their width. Water running through the wider regions travels more slowly but speeds up as it passes through the narrower parts. Your arteries are like a garden hose. If you block the end of the hose with your finger, the water's velocity increases.

If you stay in a bathtub, it causes your fingers to bloat. This is osmosis. The outermost layer of the skin swells when it absorbs water. It compensates for the increased area by wrinkling. If a dry apricot is kept in water, it is osmosis to rehydrate the fruit. When we soak resins in water, they swell up due to endosmosis. Water is drawn into the concentrated solution. This is osmosis which is basically the diffusion of water from regions of higher concentration to regions of lower concentration.

The pressure cooker uses high hydrostatic force to cook food far more quickly. We can measure the hydrostatic force in the arteries by blood pressure. The microcirculation, which supplies and drains blood from every tissue, is the terminal vascular network of the systemic circulation consisting of microvessels with diameters <20 μm. On the arterial side of the capillary, the hydrostatic pressure is high. On the venous side of the capillary, the pressure drops significantly. At this point, the oncotic pressure of the fluid within the capillary (due to the presence of salts and proteins in the blood, primarily produced by circulating albumin) pulls fluids back into the capillary.

The main functions of microcirculation are the delivery of oxygen and nutrients and the removal of carbon dioxide (CO2).

In lipoedema patients, this subtle circulation does not work. Microangiopathy has been considered as a typical histological feature of lipoedema by some researchers (Földi et al.). Microangiopathy allows red blood cells to spill more readily into the surrounding fatty tissue, resulting in bruises. Water also goes into the tissue and induces edema. Since capillaries are "leaky," this pressure forces a huge amount of fluid and nutrients into the interstitial space and tissues. They collect over and over. We see the signs of damaged circulation as edema, easily bruised skin, pain, tenderness, numbness, etc.

# VICIOUS CIRCLE

Penelope is a female character in Homer's Odyssey. She is known for her fidelity to her husband, Odysseus. Despite the attention of more than a hundred suitors during his absence, she waits twenty years for Odysseus' return.

Penelope works at weaving a shroud for the eventual funeral of her father-in-law. She tells her suitors that she will choose a husband as soon as the shroud is completed.

For Penelope, weaving becomes a form of resistance. She weaves the shroud, and every night she undoes her weaving.

It is a typical example of a vicious circle.

The worst is the vicious circle of poverty, implying that poverty is the cause of more poverty. To repay his existing debt, a poor person will borrow some more, thereby adding to his debt. This will only increase his total amount of debt.

In lipoedema, when a vicious cycle is generated, the body's homeostatic regulation is unable to break this cycle. The whole situation works in a kind of inevitable rotary way. When the circulation starts not to work properly, it leads to a vicious cycle. The disease gains momentum.

Lipoedema may cause fatigue and depression, which hinders mobility and leads to obesity. Weight gain accelerates lipoedema fat deposition, a vicious circle of weight gain. More lipoedematous fat deposition-fatigue-less mobility-more weight gain-more lipoedematous fat deposition.

Lipoedema is an inflammatory condition. Inflammation will happen, especially at the subcutaneous tissue level. Inflammation causes the proliferation of diseased tissue, which means more hypoxia due to their compression, releasing inflammatory substances, a vicious circle of inflammation-proliferation-compression-more inflammation happens. Altered fluid flux through the tissue causes the accumulation of fluid, protein, and other constituents in the interstitium, resulting in the recruitment of inflammatory cells, which stimulates fibrosis and results in difficulty in weight loss. Dysfunction of lymphatic vessels results in the accumulation of interstitial fluid (edema) in adipose tissues triggering inflammation by the recruitment of macrophages resulting in fibrosis and difficulty with weight loss. Poor circulation-fibrosis-poorer circulation-more fibrosis.

This excess fluid in the interstitial tissue will cause lipoedema fat growth (Schneider et al.) as well as hypoxia resulting in the death of adipocyte cells and macrophage recruitment. Fibrosis follows inflammation resulting in fat that is difficult to lose by exercise, diets producing caloric or ketosis, fasting, and bariatric surgery.

The excess fluid in the tissue may stimulate fat to grow, and the inflammation generated stimulates fibrosis and difficulty in weight loss. Inflammation and interstitial fluid stagnation may activate nerve fibers resulting in painful lipoedema fat tissue, and excess interstitial substance may also activate nerve fibers instigating the painful lipoedema fat tissue. Adipose tissue enlargement might not be the initial step in lipoedema patients. It might become the consequence of microvascular dysfunction, which starts a vicious cycle (Szel).

When a lipoedema patient with a painful knee starts to walk in a guarded fashion, it alters the hips' biomechanics in time. A vicious circle of painful knee-disturbed body axes-more pain in the knee.

Considering lipoedema patients have some degree of lymphocytosis due to the compression. This worsens the ongoing edema and adds further damage to their lymphatic system, placing the patient in a vicious cycle: Edema-lymphocytosis-more edema-more lymphocytosis.

Lymph stasis and edema induce tissue fibrosis and fat accumulation over time. Lymphatic vessels are dilated, and then the valves do not function properly. Inflammation decreases the degree of contraction of the lymphatic collectors and reduces the flow of lymph with an increase in swelling. Inflammation, fat deposition, and lymphatic dysfunction/lymph stasis occur as a consequence of each other in a vicious circle manner, exacerbating each other. The amount of fluid produced exceeds the transport ability of the lymphatic system during the later stages of lipoedema, and the fat tissue pressure itself induces an obstruction of the lymphatic vessels, resulting in secondary lymphedema.

Protein-rich edema deposition induces tissue fibrosis, further impairing lymphatic drainage. Therefore, at this point, the “edema” from lipoedema is likely secondary to the lymphatic pump being overloaded rather than a natural malfunction inside the lymphatics themselves. The situation is called lipolymphedema.

An intriguing hypothesis is that local inflammation of sensory nerves and adipose tissue dysfunction may act together and be responsible for the neuropathy typically found in this condition.

# KNEE PROBLEMS

The distinctive characteristics of the complex asymmetrical design of the human knee were well established more than 300 million years ago.

The knee is one of the most abused joints in the human body. It is more vulnerable to injury than other joints because it is one of the body's most mobile and flexible joints. Obesity is a primary risk factor for incident knee osteoarthritis. The potential mechanisms to link obesity and knee osteoarthritis, as biomechanical and metabolic conditions are strongly linked (Lee). Knee pain is one of the frequent symptoms of the knee in lipoedema. It can limit activity leading to lipoedema-induced obesity, which further reduces activity due to pain. They usually experience joint pain in the hips and ankles due to excessive weight of fat and fluid accumulation. A painful knee causes the patients to walk in a guarded fashion, which alters the hips' biomechanics in time. Wrongly placed stress causes wear and tear in the joints.

I sometimes see lipoedema patients who have no visible patella. It seems that fat pads around it suffocate the knee joint. After the surgery, they usually say with great surprise, "I have a knee." They come to my office during the postoperative follow-up in the third month. The first thing catching my attention is their gait. They walk in a more aesthetically pleasing way. Their walk is more energetic and more stable. Even the overpronation of their feet improves well. It is not only a great asset to their health, but it also adds to their beauty scores as well.

Over a period of time, normal posture is compromised as the body attempts to adjust to a more comfortable position when walking or at rest. This abnormal adjustment places pressure on the joints and soft tissue resulting in pain with inflammation, and the mechanical axis of the legs changes.

The bulging on the inner aspects of the thighs also impairs walking patterns. Eventually, this can result in significant orthopedic complications like, primarily valgus knee osteoarthritis.

Joint laxity can accelerate and worsen the degeneration of the joints.

Excess lipoedema fat changes the gait on the buttocks, hips, thighs, and lower legs, resulting in stress on the joints, especially the knees resulting in genu valgum (knock knees), an antalgic gait and overpronation of the feet are also induced. Gait disruption and knee pain can lead to more risk of obesity, which causes a vicious circle.

# SOCKS MARKS

Lipoedema has non-pitting edema, meaning your finger does not leave an indentation after pressing on the skin. This is not useful to diagnose the syndrome but gives important clues about the severity, lifestyle, comorbidities, medicine side effects, diet, and much more. In the later stages of lipoedema, the pitting test is positive.

The timed-pitting test gives more objective results. Check for lasting indentation if the pressure is applied to the swollen skin for about 15 seconds. This technique captures pit depth and the time needed for the skin to return to its original appearance (recovery time) as a single edema score ranging from 0 to 4.

Clinical assessments of pit depth are performed in the pretibial region of the lower leg, above the medial malleolus, behind the medial malleolus, and dorsum of the foot.

For me, socks marks are more crucial to clinical evaluation. The socks contain elastic to keep them from slipping down leave a mark. In fact, it is a test for edema. The other indentations that the leggings, pants or tight boots, and shoes leave are of clinical significance equally. The signs should be evaluated with other skin changes. The sock marks, shiny skin, and/or redness are signs of more serious problems.

Sock marks refer to clinically important edema. It is known that until the interstitial volume has increased by 2.5 to 3 liters because the tissues constituting the interstitium can easily accommodate several liters of fluid. People affected by edema often say they have trouble putting their shoes on in the evening. The feeling of heaviness in the legs is a common symptom in these patients. The heaviness in the legs is caused by the weight of the increased adipose tissue and the amount of accumulated tissue fluid.

Edema treatment is an internal part of lipoedema patients. Treatment should be guided by an underlying condition that predisposes to edema formation.

Edema has a seasonal variant in lipoedema. Heat induces peripheral blood pooling. The symptoms of edema, such as pain or heaviness, get worse in warm weather, sauna, standing for a long time, sitting for a long time, and in the evening.

Lipoedema might coexist with edema-related conditions like chronic venous problems.

When we stand up from a lying position, the microvasculature of the lower limbs constricts. This is called the veno-arterial reflex. The veno-arterial reflex prevents fluid loss to the extravascular space when the legs are dependent. Ankle edema is known as a side effect of treatment with nifedipine. According to Foldi, the veno-arteriolar reflex in lipoedema is also absent. It may be a reason for leg edema. It is a cause of swelling in people with diabetes that have neuropathy.

The complaints of lipoedema patients increase in the menstrual cycle, which is usually associated with other somatic symptoms like puffiness in the breasts and abdominal distention.

The lymphatic system that runs in parallel with the blood vascular system plays an important role in maintaining body-fluid homeostasis, immune cell trafficking, and lipid transport from the intestinal lacteals.

What is critically important is that the generation of lymph flow by intrinsic forces and the regulation of flow by both intrinsic and extrinsic forces rely on the phasic and tonic contraction of the lymphatic muscle to produce a controlled net unidirectional transport of lymph.

The edema associated with lipoedema may involve impairment of lymphatic vessels due to pressure exerted by fat tissue, which subsequently limits the inward flow of interstitial fluid.

Unlike blood, the lymphatic system is not pumped by the heart. Instead, it relies on the movement of the diaphragm, muscle contraction, skin tension, and the fluid pressures in the blood capillaries, lymphatic capillaries, and interstitial space to propel lymph fluid from across the body towards the trunk.

Lymph flow results from a complicated combination of lymph formation and intrinsic and extrinsic forces/pumps. Lymphatic pump function is very sensitive to changes in mechanical load; likely, changes in these loads on the lymphatic system of the gut are important regulators in lipid transport.

# FAINT

I examined a lipoedema patient who was around 30 years old. Although she showed the typical symptoms and appearance of lipoedema, her mother undervalued her disease and did not accept that her diagnosis was lipoedema. According to her, her daughter followed an unhealthy diet. As evidence for her thought of nonexisting lipoedema, she stated that her daughter often fainted. Referring to the secondary gains, she added her daughter had tried to avoid usual responsibilities and receive attention from their loved ones.

In the classical books of the Victorian era, women were commonly portrayed as fainting. Male authors portrayed women as weak creatures because a fragile and obedient woman is connected with a different kind of femininity. Likewise, in classical Hollywood movies, women would collapse into men's arms in melodramas (Bates).

In lipoedema patients, fainting is a common and real symptom. Vasovagal syncope is known as the most common cause of fainting. Vasovagal syncope may be triggered by pain, emotional upset, or standing too long, although a specific trigger cannot be identified frequently. It is usually preceded by prodromal symptoms of autonomic activation (sweating, pallor, nausea).

Vasovagal syncope evolved as an advantageous response to inescapable predators or stressful and possibly dangerous conditions.

The consequent slowing of the heart rate induced by vasovagal syncope may constitute a beneficial break of the cardiac pump, thereby reducing myocardial oxygen consumption. The hypothesis is presented that vasovagal fainting developed during evolution to support hemostasis. Bleeding animals with a central mechanism for the initiation of hypotension presumably had a better chance for blood clot formation and hemostasis than animals with normal blood pressure. In the context of this hypothesis, vasovagal fainting with blood or injury-displaying stimuli can be understood as an early attempt to support hemostasis before the development of larger blood losses (Diehl).

If the vasovagal reflex has persisted for millions of years along the vertebrates' evolutionary history, we can assume that it has a function and is not harmful. When it occurs associated with reducing respiratory rate, it may help to better simulate death by lessening the movements and/or sounds that accompany normal or increased heart and breathing rates that a predator can detect. It has been strongly suggested that playing dead is the right thing to do during a defensive attack. The intensity of a bear attack will decrease when the person being attacked assumes a motionless and defensive position (Herrero).

Vasovagal syncope results from a neurophysiological reflex that can be induced in most healthy people after a 30 % reduction in blood volume by venous pooling. The change to an upright position causes venous pooling of up to 800 mL of blood flow down to the legs (Hainsworth).

In lipoedema patients, one of the reasons for dizziness is orthostatic hypotension, a condition in which your blood pressure falls significantly when you stand up quickly. It intensifies in the elderly or patients with neurodegenerative diseases.

It is assumed that fainting has usually been associated with joint hypermobility syndrome, which is a condition that results in unusually supple joints and abnormally elastic blood vessels.

Gravity moves blood from the upper body to the lower limbs when standing up. As a result, there is a temporary reduction in the amount of blood in the upper body for the heart to pump (cardiac output), which decreases blood pressure. Normally, the body quickly counteracts the force of gravity and maintains stable blood pressure and blood flow. In most people, this transient drop in blood pressure goes unnoticed.

However, this transient orthostatic hypotension can cause lightheadedness that may result in falls. When signs and symptoms of orthostatic hypotension do occur, they are usually the result of a reduction in blood flow (hypoperfusion) to tissues, particularly the brain. Affected individuals may have fatigue, confusion, dizziness, blurred vision, fainting episodes (syncope), headaches, sweating, nausea, anxiety, chest pains, bowel problems, blurred vision, shaking, palpitations, and neck or shoulder pain. Symptoms are often increased in severity by warm temperatures, eating large meals, or standing for long periods.

Even the patients who did not report a history of orthostatic hypotension should be aware of this condition, which may reveal in the postoperative period or when they take off their stockings.

Lipoedema patients should be instructed to avoid triggers and drink more fluids to improve their volume status and to change positions slowly. Patients are educated about the "warning signs" of a vasovagal event and instructed to place themselves in a supine position when they feel the early symptoms so that they can neutralize gravity (Jeanmonod et al.). Dehydration worsens the condition. It would be best to drink plenty of fluids until the urine is pale yellow. They should come up from lying slowly, sitting for a while to allow the body to check its balance. The bath or shower should not be hot, which can dilate the blood vessels, leading to fluid pooling in the legs; it should be finished with cool water on the legs.

Normal functioning of the calf's venous pump is defined as the ability to maintain the venous outflow during exercise from the lower leg equal to the arterial inflow. The contraction of these muscle groups with blood expulsion into the typical collecting vein (popliteal vein) alternates rhythmically while the patient is walking. Thus, the role of lower leg muscles (calf skeletal muscles) in regulating blood pressure homeostasis while attaining an upright posture is indispensable (Masterson M. & Morgan A.). The absence of such pumping while assuming an upright posture could lead to a substantial drop in blood pressure.

# ARE FAT CELLS NEMESIS TO HUMANITY?

Fat has become "the enemy" of our modern-day society, both in the body and diet. Until the 1940s, scientists were indifferent to fat, simply characterizing it as a form of connective tissue. But in the past four decades, that view has evolved considerably. It is an endocrine organ at the center of energy homeostasis." Without it, the human body could not function properly.

From the Ottoman Era, there is a saying that a dirham (3.2 gr) of flesh covers one thousand shames. It points out the significance of adipose tissue in creating soft, curvaceous beauty.

Fat provides cushioning and insulation. It provides an excellent lubricant for the movement of the surrounding tissues. Fat protects delicate organs. It also cushions body parts exposed to high amounts of stress. Your toe and heel pads are composed of fat, and your buttocks are brimming with it. Certainly, it is an energy source, the most efficient source, yielding 9 calories per gram.

Body fat stores are the major energy stores of the body and are important determinants of survival in starvation or undernutrition. During the Ottoman Empire, arranged marriages were a part of society. Mothers chose brides in bridal ceremonies or regular Sunday baths in Hammam. They used to choose the Rubenesque girls with the hourglass figure and childbearing hips because they were more fertile. Given the multiple functions of adiposity, it is no surprise that it represents a key trait subject to sexual selection in females, who bear the direct costs of reproduction (Norgan, 1997). Across human populations, female adiposity is generally considered attractive up to a point. You can imagine what it is like to be in a Turkish bath in Ottoman Era by seeing the oil painting by Ingres. He beautifully depicts the swarming nudes from Lady Montague's letters.

There is a parallelism between choosing lipoedematous women as a mate in the Neolithic period and choosing Rubenesque women in the near past. We are genetically wired to choose partners who show signs of good fertility to maximize the chances of healthy offspring. The hourglass figure can be a measure of fertility and health. The evolution of human cognition became a sign of physical attractiveness.

It is universal to appreciate symmetry in other human physiques, as those are the translation of physically visible "good and surviving" genes. We prefer a symmetrical physique because it helps us to survive better than asymmetrical ones.

The body's symmetry is associated with developmental stability, connoting good genes, and ensuring the production of the healthiest offspring. Beauty is related to body symmetry. In that sense, lymphedema is asymmetric, which is not compatible with mate-choosing criteria, whereas lipoedema is symmetric, seen in both legs and arms.

A predominantly upper body fat distribution, commonly associated with increased visceral fat, is associated with an abnormal metabolic profile. An upper body/visceral fat distribution in obesity is strongly linked with the metabolic complications of obesity.

Because obesity is associated with diverse chronic diseases, little attention has been directed to the multiple beneficial functions of adipose tissue. Adipose tissue provides energy for growth, reproduction, and immune function and also secretes and receives diverse signaling molecules that coordinate energy allocation. Fat was once accepted as a static structure regulating lipid release and storage. After the discovery of leptin in 1994, the viewpoint towards adipose tissue was radically changed. Fat is an exocrine, endocrine, and apocrine organ and plays a role in immunity.

Fat is only one strategy for storing energy, and organisms show a wide variety of other forms of thrift, including hibernation, torpor, and a reduced activity level, along with manipulations of growth rate, body size, and relative investment in expensive organs such as brains or secondary sexual characteristics (Wells).

Gluteo-femoral fat also seems less detrimental to cardiovascular risk than central abdominal fat (Snijder et al.).

Seven out of every ten cells in fat tissue are not fat cells. According to Rosen and Spiegelman, "every gram of adipose tissue contains 1–2 million adipocytes but 4–6 million stromal vascular cells." Under obese conditions, other types of immune cells latch on to the expanding adipocytes, contributing to insulin resistance and chronic low-level inflammation.

One day, one of my patients told me she felt like her fats took control of her mind and kept saying, "eat, eat, more eat."

The more fat tissue the body has, the more calories are locked away in this fat tissue, leaving fewer calories in the bloodstream to meet your body's energy requirements. These fat cells then steal your calories (Ludwig and Friedman). The more fat we have, the more we need to eat because the body needs more and more calories. This shift cannot be achieved by dieting only. As long as these fat cells remain in your body, they will continue to steal calories away for storage.

This reminds me of a famous Russian novel. Goncharov portrayed the prototype of a fat and lazy man in that book. The central character, Oblomov, rarely leaves his room or bed. He conducts most of his daily business from his bed. It is a quote from the novel. "When you don't know what you're living for, you don't care how you live from one day to the next."

# HORMONE WARS

The condition occurs almost exclusively in women and usually starts or worsens during puberty, pregnancy, or menopause. The incidence rises in women who have external estrogen treatment and in vitro fertilization. They all provide solid evidence that it is largely influenced and triggered by sex hormones. Estrogen is known to modulate lipid metabolism in white adipose tissue directly. Although estrogen is a major trigger of lipoedema, insulin, cortisol, and thyroid hormone deficiency contribute to this condition.

When progesterone and estrogen are at adequate levels in the body, the body will run optimally; however, it is when estrogen becomes too high (or progesterone gets too low) a woman will find herself in a state of "estrogen dominance," which can disrupt several bodily functions.

When adequate levels of progesterone do not balance estrogen levels, women tend to retain more fluid than usual. Breast discomfort, swelling, mood swings, headaches, fatigue, difficulty sleeping, hair loss, weight gain, bloating, and a decrease are some of the other symptoms. Progesterone is a natural anti-inflammatory. It lowers insulin levels; it is a natural diuretic and can significantly reduce bloating and swelling.

Estrogen dominance results from a complex imbalance that does not usually occur overnight. Your body often produces too much estrogen and not enough progesterone.

Insulin promotes lipogenesis, and insulin resistance worsens edema formation; a diet avoiding glycemic and insulin peaks and allowing adequate intervals between meals (i.e., an isoglycemic diet) may be desirable in lipoedema. Even small increases in plasma insulin dramatically suppress adipose tissue lipolysis.

Insulin is affected by hormone imbalance, and estrogen dominance can lead to excess insulin release. Increases in insulin can lead to sugar cravings that can be hard to control. This is why many women crave chocolate or other sweets during premenstrual syndrome.

During evolution, the fluctuations in environmental conditions demanded an adaptation for human survival. Climate, seasonal, and vegetation conditions forced the human species to develop a flexible metabolism. Humans' metabolism was shaped by adaptation to a broader range of different food sources (biodiversity), abundant daily exercise frequently under fasting conditions (foraging behavior), as well as unpredictable food supply (intermittent fasting), depending on the daily foraging success. The basic metabolic programs of humans' primal hunter-gatherer lifestyle are opposed to the current sedentary lifestyle with the constant availability of energy-dense but nutrient-deficient foods. Our adaptive mechanism becomes maladaptive in the current environment. A dynamic of feast and famine characterized our relationship with food. Evolution seems to have shaped the human metabolic system for ancient times of frequent energy deficiency rather than the present opulence, which entails adverse consequences, such as hyperglycemia, hyperinsulinemia, dyslipidemia, and a chronic proinflammatory state induced by, among other things, accumulating visceral body fat. The modern lifestyle promotes the continuous fueling of adipocytes. In response to adipose hypertrophy, neutrophils, macrophages, natural killer cells, and other immune cells infiltrate adipose tissue and develop an inflammatory environment in the further process.

Insulin resistance is a condition in which cells in your muscles, fat, and liver exhibit reduced response to insulin. This is accompanied by increased insulin synthesis from your pancreas resulting in hyperinsulinemia which is thought to be a compensatory response to reduced insulin sensitivity. A preliminary diagnostic criterion for insulin resistance is high levels of plasma insulin in relation to glucose levels. Insulin resistance evolved as a physiologically adaptive mechanism in human survival, and the same mechanism is inappropriately activated on a chronic basis in the current environment, leading to the manifestations of metabolic syndrome.

For approximately 99.5% of our existence, we lived as hunter-gatherers being metabolically prepared for any kind of environmental condition. Human survival has relied upon the ability to withstand starvation through energy storage, the capacity to fight off infection by a proinflammatory immune response, and the ability to cope with physical stressors by an adaptive stress response. Energy storage, mainly as glycogen in the liver and triglycerides in adipose tissue, is regulated by the anabolic actions of insulin. On the other hand, mobilization of stored energy during infection, trauma, or stress is served by the temporary inhibition of insulin action (insulin resistance) in target tissues by proinflammatory cytokines and stress hormones. In the current environment, high energy intake, low physical activity, and chronic stress favor surplus fat storage in adipose tissue depots, far exceeding their storage capacity and liporegulation (Tsatsoulis et al.).

Apparently, since evolution is a slow-acting process, modern humans are not yet well adapted to a sedentary lifestyle. Nowadays, hunting and gathering need only a few steps into the kitchen or a short drive to the local food store, which implies substantial energy intake by no or less energy expenditure of the locomotor system.

Food-seeking behavior is an evolutionary-based motivational drive to forage in order to maintain energy balance on a homeostatic level. Foraging success in the form of food represents the primal reward for a physical effort. In order to avoid overnutrition, our metabolic homeostatic system involves several hormonal regulators of hunger and satiety, such as leptin, ghrelin, and insulin, which act on hypothalamic and brainstem circuits to inhibit further feeding. Dysfunction of this homeostatic system can result in a persistent state of positive energy balance, overeating, and obesity. Palatable high-caloric foods might be a major reason for this dysfunction in the Western world by exchanging the regulation of food intake from homeostatic to rewarding pathways.

Most of my patients are diagnosed with thyroid insufficiency. Although science has not shown solid evidence of the link between lipoedema and thyroid insufficiency, it is quite obvious clinically. Even mild thyroid dysfunction in the form of subclinical hypothyroidism is linked to significant changes in body weight.

The thyroid gland does not seem to be affected in a small group of patients. In low levels of progesterone seen in lipoedema patients, the liver produces excess amounts of a protein called thyroid-binding globulin. This thyroid-binding globulin binds to the thyroid hormones, inhibiting the hormones from being used properly by your body. The net effect of this is a form of hypothyroidism that some refer to as type 2 hypothyroidism, which does not appear on blood tests since the problem is within your cells rather than in your blood.

Most of my patients shared the information with me that a ketogenic diet, including healthy fats, was more beneficial for losing weight. Fish or omega-3 supplementation, avocados, olive oil, and nuts might be related to increased adiponectin levels. More fiber supplementation would be more effective in increasing its levels. Exercise also increases adiponectin levels.

Adiponectin protects the vascular endothelium and facilitates the proper metabolism of glucose and lipids. High concentrations have been documented in cases of longevity. Low concentrations of adiponectin cause insulin resistance. Adiponectin also acts as a vasodilatory and anti-inflammatory factor. Low levels of this protein correlate with impaired vasodilation, thus impeding microcirculation. These findings imply a probable link between low adiponectin concentrations and cellulite development.

Leptin is also synthesized by adipocytes. Leptin levels are positively correlated with obesity, insulin resistance, and increased risk of cardiovascular events. Several studies have confirmed the relationship between hyperleptinemia and endothelial dysfunction. Adiponectin and leptin work antagonistically, and their concentrations reflect the present metabolic state.

At daytime, leptin levels decrease, and hunger signals emerge to increase sensitivity to brain reward systems, which boost the motivational drive of physical activity, facilitating foraging behavior. In contrast, leptin levels increase during nighttime since appetite needs to be reduced to avoid disturbing sleep by hunger signals.

The fastest release of adiponectin, produced by adipocytes as a fundamental signal for the brain to modulate food intake, occurs at 10 a.m., synonymous with the greatest glucose tolerance. Accordingly, it seems contradictory that high glycemic foods are recommended for breakfast to provide energy for a sedentary daily routine since cortisol has generated energy at sunrise for more than 2.5 million years without energy intake.

# BROWN ADIPOSE TISSUE AND ITS THERAPEUTIC POTENTIAL

Adipose tissue is the primary site of storage for excess energy. Still, it serves as an endocrine organ capable of synthesizing a number of biologically active compounds that regulate metabolic homeostasis.

Two main types of adipose tissue in our body, white adipose tissue and brown adipose tissue, may coexist throughout the adipose tissue sites. Brown adipose tissue is essential to dissipate energy through the regulation of thermogenesis. The function of brown adipose tissue is to transfer energy from food into heat.

Human infants possess abundant brown adipose tissue at birth, accounting for 1.4% of the total body. Brown adipose tissue plays a critical role in thermoregulation in infants and young children. Brown adipose tissue grows in size and masses until adolescence, after which it gradually recedes until old age. Impaired brown adipose tissue development in the human infant has been implicated in the high mortality rates of preterm infants. Genes that augment brown adipose tissue function would be highly advantageous in cold climates. Endothermy (regulating body temperature by metabolic means) is characterized by high metabolic rates. The ability of active brown fat to expend high amounts of energy has raised interest in stimulating thermogenesis therapeutically to treat metabolic diseases related to obesity.

# CELLULITIS, CELLULITE, AND SKIN BARRIER

The term “cellulitis” is often confused with” cellulite “; the former refers to a potentially serious infection of the deeper layers of skin, and the next is used for orange peel skin.

Cellulitis presents itself with the four classical signs of infection rubor (redness), dolor (pain), tumor (swelling), and calor (heat), still the same as recorded initially by Celsus in the 1st century A.D.

The Epic of Gilgamesh, which deals with such eternal human problems as sickness, old age, death, and fame, is regarded as the oldest written story on Earth. In the Gilgamesh tablet XI, Gilgamesh obtains the magic plant that will make him young again. Unfortunately, it is eaten by a serpent that sheds its old skin as it departs and replaces it with a new shiny one, apparently reborn.

It reminds the desquamation phenomena of dead cells shedding from the skin in a repeated cycle of 4-6 weeks. This oversimplifying process was accepted without biological activity and function until recently gained importance. This pile of dead cells makes it possible to discharge the potentially detrimental materials from the skin without retaining them.

These dead cells, the lipid matrix holding them together, and antimicrobial peptides provide a crucial protective barrier from environmental irritants and harmful microbes, as well as the unregulated loss of water and solutes. Thermal and ultraviolet barrier function and the initiation of inflammation through cytokine activation are just some of its other functions.

This skin barrier is at high risk in lipoedema patients because swollen skin tends to compromise that barrier, leading to subsequent infection. Protein-rich fluid, particularly in advanced stages, provides a perfect medium for microbial growth. In addition, particularly deep folds and crevices harbor bacteria.

The stagnation of lymph limits the clearance of bacteria, resulting in an ineffective defense against infection, and a decrease in local immunity increases the cellulitis risk. Bacteria eliminated by phagocytosis are effectively cleared through lymphatic drainage. In lymphedema patients, the accumulated bacterial toxins in lymphatic tissue cannot be drained sufficiently, causing systemic symptoms due to cytokine release.

While I examine a lipoedema patient, I always pay extra attention to foot hygiene, toenail problems like fungus, hallus valgus deformities, cracking/ fissuring of the skin barrier, provides a portal of entry, increasing the risk of cellulitis through invasion by microorganisms via an opportunistic pathway.

Cellulitis is a potentially dangerous bacterial infection that affects the deeper layers of the skin and may spread to the connective tissue. The bacteria that cause cellulitis can cause considerable damage to the deeper skin layers. Cellulitis is common in the arms and legs but can also occur in other places on the body or face.

Untreated cellulitis can spread to the deep tissues, even leading to blood poisoning or death of the affected tissue. Therefore, cellulitis infections must be treated at once after symptoms of rash, itching, redness, pain, increased skin temperature, swelling, fever, or flu-like symptoms are important for swollen legs.

A higher incidence of cellulitis with lymphangitis was demonstrated in patients with lower-extremity lymphedema, weakened immune system, obesity, smoking, alcohol consumption, and diabetes mellitus. The immune system may become weaker due to certain medications, including the drugs that suppress the body's immune response.

Lymphangitic streaking, characterized by linear erythema on the skin, is most commonly observed in the setting of bacterial infection. Noninfectious lymphangitic streaking may also occur after bites from various insects, ticks, and spiders.

Lipoedema patients should avoid causing damage to their delicate skin; the infection even occurs after an unnoticed small wound, bad nail care, toe web maceration, and tinea pedis.

In our culture, leech therapy and cubbing are quite popular for the edematous legs. They certainly add extra risk.

Lipoedema patients should not use cosmetics that irritate their skin. The acid protection layer of the skin must not be damaged. The skin must not be dry or cracked. They should not use alkaline soap; use a soap with an acid pH value.

Cellulite is currently considered an endocrine-metabolic micro-circulatory disorder. The change in the skin topography is only the tip of the iceberg. The first step in cellulite treatment is simulating microcirculation and removing accumulated fluids and toxic elements.

Rubens aestheticizes orange peel skin in his paintings. The Fur is a portrait by Rubens of his second wife getting out of the bath. The existence of leg cellulitis is quite apparent.

He also painted cellulitis in the back of Venus in front of the Mirror, dents on the buttocks, and in the legs of "The Three Graces," It seems that cellulite was a part of post-pubertal women, even as the ideal of beauty. It was considered a cosmetic problem in modern times but until recently. Now we discuss its relationship with metabolism problems.

Why has cellulite become a female nemesis recently? Dysfunction of adipocytes leads to changes in skin topography. What we see on the skin is the sign of an underlying metabolic problem.

An improper and sedentary lifestyle speeds up the condition. Excessive intake of food products rich in fats, with a high salt and preservative content, has been associated with the development of various metabolic disorders, including hyperinsulinemia, a condition that can increase lipodystrophy. A sedentary lifestyle plays a similar role. Hormonal disturbances, genetic factors, and lipoedema also predispose women to develop cellulite. Poor physical activity adds up to the condition by affecting microcirculation.

Some patients visiting my office point out their overweight husbands and explain why they do not have cellulitis. They take it as unfair to women. In the superficial part of adipose, the collagen fibers lie perpendicular to the skin surface. The slightest amount of excess fat in this layer results in bulging outwards. Fibrous septae architecture that compartmentalizes the adipose tissue is quite different in females than males.

Lipoedema fat like a lack of oxygen. The contraction of small blood vessels impairs the local microcirculation resulting in lipodystrophy. Combined cigarette smoking with alcohol consumption, their negative effects are doubled. Alcohol stimulates lipogenesis and causes body dehydration, resulting in excessive and improper fat storage.

Estrogen shapes women's bodies as the brush of nature. Excessive quantities of estrogen distort the painting. It increases wall permeability, which may lead to the swelling of the surrounding tissues. Excessive relaxation of the veins is observed, causing blood stasis and resulting in swelling, ischemia, and hypoxia in the subcutaneous tissue.

Some patients say that they cannot lose weight from their thighs or buttocks. Are we lipoedema patients? Abdominal fat cells are more responsive to catecholamines than femoral and gluteal fat cells (Maurigie). Fat cells in the buttocks, thigh, and knees have a greater proportion of fat-storing alpha receptors than fat cells located elsewhere in the body.

It means that you lose little weight in these regions when you lose weight, but you gain weight, and most of the fat accumulates in these regions.

# FLAT FOOT AS EVOLUTIONARY MISMATCH

Our ancestors were running outside in nature, exposing bare feet to sand, grass, and dirt. Until relatively recently, all humans were either barefoot or wore minimal footwear, lacking cushioning and arch supports; this gave our feet the proprioceptive training necessary to build strong and durable arches.

For the evolution of bipedalism, stiff feet are of the essence. What are stiff feet? While walking or running walk, our feet maintain their shapes without severely bending despite pushing on the ground with force exceeding several times the body's weight. This is unique to humans, enabling us to walk and run effectively on the ground using two feet. There are two main arches of the foot. The longitudinal arch runs from heel to forefoot.

The arch and tissues create a bow-and-string structure considered the main source of the foot's stiffness for nearly a century. The foot has a second arch that runs across the width of the midfoot, known as the transverse arch. Our arched foot, which is not a characteristic of other primates, is a unique feature crucial for human bipedalism. The arch also retains sufficient flexibility to store and release mechanical energy like a spring.

In the ancient town of Ephesus, you can see the magnificent ruins of the ancient world, like the Library of Celsus. Education was much valued, and through the cult of Artemis, the city became a bastion of women's rights and a place for female artists. One of the things attracting my attention is a pictogram representing a flat foot engraved into the Marble Road. According to the arch index, a highly reliable test, this flat foot is the oldest known illustration of this particular pathology (Wokaunn M et al.). It is a mystery why a flat foot was used in a pictogram. The rarity of a metal or a gemstone determines whether it is classified as precious. Was it because flat foot was rarely seen and therefore taken as exceptional?

Bulky and padded shoes with sturdy arch supports, flip-flops, and high heels shoes have negatively impacted how our feet interact with the ground and changed the biomechanics of our gait. High heels shorten the Achilles tendon and limit dorsiflexion. Flip-flops impair the windlass mechanism. Arch supports limit proprioceptive input while weakening the intrinsic musculature and ligaments that naturally keep the arch strong. Modern shoes reduce the role of the foot muscles in maintaining arch stiffness, thereby leading to less growth and possibly even atrophy through disuse.

Most individuals diagnosed with flat foot have a 'flexible' flat foot, characterized by substantial eversion of the rear foot during weight-bearing, resulting in a marked drop in longitudinal height and reduced longitudinal height stiffness during walking. Although this condition is often asymptomatic, it might cause foot pain and fatigue after standing for long periods.

Reduced longitudinal arch stiffness is also a risk factor for numerous lower extremity musculoskeletal disorders, including plantar fasciitis, knee osteoarthritis, tibialis posterior tendinopathy, and metatarsal stress fracture.

The reduction in longitudinal arch stiffness that characterizes flat foot is a mismatch condition caused by the human foot being inadequately adapted to the novel environmental condition of wearing shoes that provide comfort and protection at the expense of weaker foot muscles.

Wolf's Law states that our bodies will adapt to the loads under which they are placed. Sitting all day and wearing over-padded or heeled shoes removes the beneficial stress from our foot's intrinsic muscles. If we walk around with collapsed arches, some work must be done to correct that. A properly functioning foot arch should be a flexible high dome that can flatten a little, but not completely, when walking. It's supported by four layers of muscles and more than a dozen ligaments. Walking or running transfers weight to the big toe in the push-off phase of gait. This transfer of energy through the kinetic chain needs to flow unimpeded. With a collapsed arch, energy, and torque bleed from the system into other body areas unsuited to handle such loads, including the medial structures of the knee joint.

As stated by Leonardo da Vinci, "The human foot is a masterpiece of engineering and a work of art." This nature's ultimate piece of art even supports all body weight on the tips of fully extended feet within pointed shoes in ballerinas. Flatfoot is a condition in which the longitudinal arch of the foot is lost. Look at your footprint when you step into sand or out of a pool. If it looks like a rectangle, your natural arch is nonexistent in a weight-bearing position. This overpronation is likely to cause many biomechanical faults in the human body, starting at the foot and going all the way up to the cervical spine and temporomandibular joint. Because of flat feet, many people commonly experience pain in their heel, knee, hip, low back, and cervical spine.

When you drop an object, it simply falls to the ground. We don't think much about the force behind it at all. Gravity, whose effects are so deeply entrenched in our everyday lives, even lipoedema. The benefits of gravity and acceleration on the musculoskeletal and cardiovascular systems are obvious. Bone loss and muscle atrophy are the negative effects of reduced gravity in space. The regulation of fluid volume is heavily influenced by gravity. As astronauts experience free fall, the fluids shift to the upper part of the body, and astronauts have puffy heads.

The swelling in lipoedema is dependent edema caused by the effects of gravity and occurs when fluid accumulates in the lower parts of the body.

There is one important but not well-known structure that certainly deserves admiration in the foot, which struggles against gravity. The plantar venous pump is a network of capillaries that promotes lymphatic and venous return upward when compressed during walking and running. A plantar vault with three arches and the plantar fascia acting like a bouncy trampoline help to get it worked properly. Suppose you squeeze your feet into very tight shoes. Its functionality becomes limited and adapts to the new situation. This venous pump of the human foot is the first step in venous return from the lower extremity to the heart.

I always ask my patients for the presence of flat feet. If it exists, proper shoes should be made before the surgery. These patients have a walking pattern of foot slaps. They slap down their feet with each step from the ankle rather than striking with the heel and rolling through a step, pushing off with the toe. In flat foot patients, it may be proposed that blood pooling in the veins will occur due to the ineffective use of a plantar venous pump.

Interestingly, larger lower leg muscles in persons with flat feet may enhance the muscle pump action of the leg and facilitate venous return to the heart. Flat feet require a different balance of muscle strength to maintain strength and stability by compensating for changes in foot structure.

Proper calf muscle function is one of the most significant factors outflowing of venous blood from the lower extremities. Failure of the muscle or venous pump in lipoedema seems to be the most underestimated pathophysiological factor.

Orthopedic problems are very common in patients with lipoedema. The loss of the inner arches of the feet is common in patients with hypermobility; the arches cannot resist the body weight due to the weak ligaments, leading to the collapse of the arch. They contribute progression of edema because they prevent fluid transportation from the feet. Flat feet should be analyzed and treated with adequate shoes. A proper shoe should provide cushioning, comfortable arch support, control pronation, and reduce foot friction. These patients are strongly recommended to add special exercises to their daily routines. If there is localized fat accumulation in the inner thigh or inner knee, they can hinder mobility and have priority to treatment.

Having flat feet can also cause the appearance of out-toeing. Out-toeing can make a child look like they're waddling from side to side. Parents may notice that their child's shoes wear out or have more noticeable scuff marks on the outer edges of the shoes. Lipoedema patients with reduced ankle mobility adopt a shuffling type of gait, not heel-to-toe walking. After liposuction, I noticed that normal walking is restored and regained in most patients.

There is an inspirational African story. It is said that a man ventured into the inhospitable lands of Africa. Only his porters accompanied him. They each carried a machete in their hands and made their way through the thick vegetation. They crossed a river. They walked up a hill. The porters suddenly stopped. The explorer was surprised. They had only been walking for a few hours. So, he asked them: "Why have we stopped? Are you already tired after just a few hours of walking?" Then one of the porters looked at him and said: "No sir, we are not tired. We have been moving very quickly, so our souls are left behind. Now we must wait for them to catch up with us again."

This story summarizes the whole problem of evolutionary maladaptation. Cultural evolution is indeed faster than biological evolution. Our stone age bodies have not adapted to modern conditions.

# VENOUS PROBLEMS: ANOTHER ADAPTATION PROBLEM

Humanity faced certain diseases, first after the Neolithic Revolution and second after the Industrial Revolution. The disease of varicose veins is among the typical mismatch diseases. The incidence is very much lower in preindustrial communities. It has been assumed that they are a disease of maladaptation (John Powles). When the relationship between human beings and the natural world is so rapid, it renders biological adaptation extremely difficult.

Chronic venous insufficiency is a disease that affects up to one-third of the population. It is related to a deficiency of dietary fiber, creator carbohydrates, and caloric intake. There is also a positive relationship between sedentary activities (standing or sitting) and the presence of varicose veins.

Cultural change has outpaced genetic adaptation to such an extent that there is now discordance between our Paleolithic pre-agricultural hunter-gatherer genotype and many features of our present lifestyle. The Western diet is likely deficient in a number of micronutrients essential for the integrity of the vein wall.

The superficial venous systems are the great saphenous and small saphenous veins, often used in bypass surgery. Any veins above the deep muscular fascia, which are not deep veins, are considered superficial veins. The superficial venous system drains the blood flow from the skin and the subcutaneous tissues.

The great saphenous vein is the longest vein in the body. It originates on the medial side of the foot and ascends anterior to the medial malleolus and then along the medial side of the calf and thigh and drains into the common femoral vein.

The saphenofemoral junction is critical in understanding flow patterns, treatment approaches, and the recurrence of varicosities.

The deep venous system is responsible for approximately 90% of the venous blood flow in the lower extremities.

Muscle contractions make a vein pump the venous blood flowing upwards during walking. The calf muscle pump is called the peripheral heart. During ambulation, the calf muscle pump empties the venous system, and the veins' pressure decreases. Relaxation of the muscle pump then allows blood to refill to the deep venous system.

Perforators are bridging channels between the superficial and deep venous systems. These veins obliquely perforate the deep fascia and play a key role in equilibrating blood flow during calf muscle contraction because of valves that prevent reflux from the deep venous system to the superficial venous system.

As components of the vascular system, spider veins and vascular changes in lipoedema patients also suggest a level of microangiopathy (disease of the small blood vessels). The coupling of these results would suggest that lipoedema may be driven by vascular issues that manifest in the increased edema buildup and subsequent limitations of fluid removal from the interstitial space.

Free radicals damage the microvasculature, leading to increased permeability. This free radical damage is countered by the body's antioxidant system, which is dependent primarily on a wide range of vitamins and other phytochemicals found in fruit and vegetables. A number of these plant-derived substances are well known and include ascorbic acid, tocopherol, and bioflavonoids.

It has been shown that flavonoids are able to suppress the formation of free radicals. Flavonoids are a diverse group of compounds and are responsible for the colors of fruits and vegetables. Over four thousand flavonoids have been classified according to chemical structure.

Varicose veins are dilated, bulging, superficial veins measuring at least 3 mm in diameter that become progressively more tortuous and enlarged. Cutaneous changes include skin hyperpigmentation, stasis dermatitis, and ulceration. They cause pain if superficial thrombophlebitis develops.

Stockings with compression pressure between 20 and 30 mmHg are recommended for patients with varicose veins with or without edema (C2 to C3). Stockings between 30 and 40 mmHg pressure are recommended for patients with advanced venous skin change or an ulcer (C4 to C6).

Telangiectasis, reticular veins, small varicose veins, and venous segments with reflux can be treated with sclerotherapy.

Varicose veins are not only a cosmetic issue but also can cause problems like heavy legs or cramps in the lower legs. The symptoms of lipoedema and venous insufficiency are similar. They both cause heaviness, tenderness, fatigue, and swelling. These symptoms usually get worse towards the end of the day. Warm weather, sitting or standing for long periods, worsens the symptoms. Obviously, the symptoms will be doubled in case of the coexistence of both diseases.

Reticular veins have a diameter of less than 3 mm and are often tortuous and located in the subdermal or subcutaneous tissue (Eklof; Porter).

The cause is unknown. Patients may be asymptomatic or can report pain, burning, or itching. Risk factors include family history, pregnancy, local trauma, and hormonal factors (Goldman).

Telangiectasias, or spider veins, are dilated venules or arterioles (small superficial veins) measuring less than 1.0 mm in diameter.

The presence of telangiectasias may be associated with insufficiency of major venous systems; 50% to 62% of insufficient perforating veins are found in the presence of telangiectasias (Andrade 2009). They can occur on their own (primary), after skin injury like sun damage, or may arise due to an underlying condition (secondary).

Interestingly, the appearance of the varicose veins does not always indicate how severe the symptoms are. I sometimes see patients with very large and bumpy veins with no discomfort.

I sometimes observe the disappearance of some varicose veins after liposuction, which astonish the patients. In fact, a similar situation occurs for various postpartum veins. Because there is no research on this observation, it would be better to review the result of research performed for pregnancy and various veins.

Hormonal aspects and hormonal pattern variations have important implications in dilatation and determining decreased venous wall tone during pregnancy. The other factor is weight gain – which makes it harder for the blood in their leg veins to flow back to the heart properly, and the compression of the uterus on iliac veins plays a role in the genesis of “pregnancy” varicosities.

Postpartum or “pregnancy” veins usually go away within several months after pregnancy. After six months, most minor vein dilatations (visible at the end of pregnancy) may become almost invisible and clinically irrelevant. If a postpartum varicose vein is not reduced in size between six and twelve months after delivery, it will likely remain and eventually progress. Most vein size and visibility improvements occur within twelve months of the end of pregnancy. The disappearance of most veins after the end of the pregnancy may also be a consequence of hormonal changes associated with improved hemodynamics at the level of intra-abdominal veins. Postpartum varicose veins tend, at least partially, to regain their normal functions and shapes, as seen in several studies using compression. Regaining tone and muscular functions, most dilated or varicose veins may regress to the almost original shape and size.

In lipoedema patients, some of the varicose veins are reduced in size or disappear between six and twelve months after liposuction. It may be attributed to the improvement in circulation, decrease of fluid overload, weight loss, a decrease of inflammation, and of course, the support with compressive stockings helps the varicose veins regain their tone. Generally, it is better to delay invasive treatments for a few months (up to 6–9 months) to avoid treating veins that may spontaneously regress.

# ELEVATION

In lipoedema, elevation is recommended for reducing edema. The elevation is not simply to put your feet up on things like the cowboys putting their feet up tables in Hollywood movies. The foot should be above the hip with a fully supported bent knee. The patients usually say that their legs are quite thin in the morning but gradually get larger over the day. Obviously, gravity leads to an increase of venous pressure in the dependent legs, particularly in patients with venous insufficiency. If patients say their edema quickly disappears when they lie down and elevate the legs, the edema is caused by fluid accumulation, not lymph stasis.

In lipoedema patients, different sources of edema. Filtration edema caused by venous overloading will tend to improve by 90% or more with overnight elevation, but edema due to lymph collection will improve by only 10–20% at best. Lymph drainage can be improved using simple physiological principles to stimulate lymph flow.

My patients with loose tissue often complain of edema. It might be attributed to more vascular damage in such patients showing the problem of collagen production. A mechanical factor also exists. In lipoedema patients with loose tissue, edema continues to accumulate in large volumes. In patients with tight skin, fewer edema symptom is observed. Stiffness of tissues resists swelling. Compressive stocking will be a wise approach to mimic tissue stiffness, adding extra resistance to the tissue. Patients who work in a sitting position often complain about edema. A pressure 'graduation' of compression stockings, which is higher in the distal than in the proximal segments of the leg, is recommended.

# PALEOLITHIC NUTRITION: FACT OR MYTH

Lipoedema is not caused by nutrition and, therefore, cannot be influenced by diets, and there is no specific diet to cure lipoedema. Lipoedema is not only a simple enlargement of the fat cells but also a change in the structure of the fatty tissue. For this reason, the disease cannot be influenced by weight loss. Their family members and, unfortunately, doctors and dietitians often tell them that their disease is the result of the wrong nutrition. Although the effects and success of specific diets differ from patient to patient, the leg circumference is little affected. Weight loss should not be achieved at the expense of muscle mass which worsens the symptoms. A strict diet makes the organism change to low flame so that the subsequent "normal" eating habits when resumed, leading to a sudden increase in weight. They can lose weight with a calorie-restricted diet. Still, it has minimal effect on abnormal body fat distribution, resulting in eating disorders, increased obesity risk, depression, and other psychological complaints.

The number of fat cells in our bodies is set during adolescence and remains constant through adulthood, regardless of whether you gain or lose weight. Therefore, it can be so hard for some people to lose weight and keep them off. Because the number of fat cells is fixed, they can only get bigger when we put on weight.

Although dietetic strategies cannot prevent the disproportional fat distribution, they may reduce local inflammation, thus ameliorating symptoms and improving general well-being and overall health. Besides, it helps the patient take control of lipoedema after liposuction.

A one-size-fits-all diet approach is problematic. Dietary recommendations should be individualized for each patient. There is a plethora of anecdotal report from some lipoedema patients regarding the positive effects of different diets on the internet. Since anecdotal evidence is collected casually or formally and relies entirely on personal testimony, they play a minor role in science. To incorporate anecdotes into medical evidence, they should be documented from a scientific perspective.

The fundamental argument behind the Paleo diet is that Today's people have not adapted to the present day's diet they follow. Our bodies still behave like those of our hunter-gatherer ancestors. The hunter-gatherers ate nuts, seeds, fruits, coarse vegetables, fish, and lean meat while excluding grains and dairy products. The way of life of hunter-gatherers was as varied as the many environments in which they lived: tundra, valleys, seaside, tropical rainforests, and more, such that no single "Paleodiet" existed.

It is a fallacy that our ancient ancestors were mainly carnivores. They mostly ate a plant-based diet. The diet was broad and heavily influenced by geographical location and food availability. It is also not true that hunters and gatherers did not eat any carbohydrates at all. The 'paleo diet' concept is used to justify low-carbohydrate diets. Our understanding of hunter-gather lifeways has significant limitations. Carbohydrates like honey have been part of their diet. Diets in hunter-gatherers tend to be less energy dense and richer in fiber and micronutrients than modern diets but are not invariably low in carbohydrates, as sometimes argued. Our bodies use carbohydrates for fuel during aerobic exercises, such as walking. Without adequate carbohydrates in the diet, our body turns to both body fat and muscle for energy. This results in the breaking down of muscle mass, which is known to increase our metabolism and help us burn more calories daily. Feelings of physical fatigue and exhaustion throughout the day and during exercise can be signs of muscle breakdown.

They lived off of what nature provided. What they ate depended on what they could find each season, eating fruit and berries when they ripened. It might give a clue that we should eat seasonally.

Clearly, “Stone Age” humans ate a variety of high-quality foods rich in nutrients and fiber. Modern diets provide much less variety than this diet and are loaded with artificial sugars and salt. Because game animals are highly lean, hunter-gatherers eat much less saturated fat than Western cultures and generally eat more polyunsaturated than saturated fat. They did not eat processed foods containing additives, pesticides, herbicides, or other potentially toxic agricultural chemicals. In addition, hunter-gatherers eat an enormous variety of wild plants. In contrast, in modern societies, only a small proportion of plants make up the bulk of the food supply, with the most significant percentage contributed by cereal grains.

From a realistic point of view, it is impossible to replicate the exact diet that our Paleolithic ancestors ate. Food consumed in the Paleo Diet was dramatically different than that of today. We have selectively bred to produce higher yields, to taste sweeter. Domesticated livestock has a high-fat content compared to wild prey.

The fruits or vegetables they consumed did not include pesticides or hormones (Figure 8). Today, you cannot find the same fruit even if it does not contain pesticides and is purely organic, produced by an heirloom seed. Even fresh fruits produced organically are stored in refrigerators or cold storage. They lose their taste and aroma. In some areas of Anatolia, you can see the fig trees alongside the narrow paths owned by nobody. You cannot find them in the markets because they grow themselves; when you pick a fig from its branch, you witness a miracle. Dense milk from the branch comes out. You can taste the freshest fruit in the world. It is still alive; it is not only full of nutrition, but it is also full of life energy. Hunter-Gatherers ate the fruits they picked from branches and witnessed the miracles of nature, which helped them keep connecting with nature.

I do not want to paint a pessimistic picture of the situation. We can do our best to follow their paleo diets, but not much of it Without romanticizing that era, a diet that mimics the nutritional characteristics of diets in the Paleolithic era would be a wise approach. The good news is that we should focus on a modern version of Paleolithic life.

Preliminary studies using a contemporary diet based on Paleolithic food groups (meat, fish, shellfish, fresh fruits and vegetables, roots, tubers, eggs, and nuts) revealed promising results, including favorable changes in risk factors, such as weight, waist circumference, C-reactive protein, HbA1c, blood pressure, glucose tolerance, insulin secretion, insulin sensitivity and lipid profiles (Blomquist C et al.). A Paleolithic diet decreased lipogenesis-promoting factors, improved insulin sensitivity, and reduced circulating triglycerides.

The primary difference between the popular paleo diets and other healthy diets is the absence of whole grains and legumes, considered good sources of fiber, vitamins, and other nutrients. Also absent from the diet are dairy products, which are good sources of protein and calcium. There is evidence that human biochemistry can adjust to suit changes in diet over a relatively short time. For example, about forty percent of the world population has, it seems, developed the ability to digest lactose (cow's milk) more efficiently than our ancestors. So, the idea that humans are naturally unable to deal with grains and other recent foods is not well founded. For most people, staying committed to any diet that is too restrictive of one or more food categories is very difficult.

The most extensively studied tribe is the Hadza tribe from central Tanzania because the African continent is considered the hallmark of human evolution. The Hadza group resides in the tropical forest, and their diet mainly consists of plants, fruits, tubers, and game animals. One of the most popular food groups for them is honey. The Hadza tend to maintain the same healthy weight, body mass index, and walking speed throughout their adult lives. Their diet consists of various types of meat, vegetables, fruits, and a significant amount of honey. In fact, they get 15 to 20 percent of their calories from honey, a simple carbohydrate. A natural diet and high levels of physical activity clearly contribute to the enviable health of hunter-gatherers.

There are a few things to adapt to a modern lifestyle. They do not eat refined sugar, which is absorbed rapidly into the bloodstream; our bodies are not well-programmed to handle it efficiently. An abrupt rise in blood glucose levels may trigger the pancreas to release an excessive amount of insulin, which can lead to reactive hypoglycemia and a compensatory increase in blood sugar levels–raising compounds such as epinephrine and cortisol.

Fire control has had a major impact on the course of human evolution. It has also influenced human biology, assisting in providing a high-quality diet that has fueled the increase in brain size through the Pleistocene. Fire allowed people to cook their food, thus expanding their source of nutrition to less digestible or tasty plants. Cooking greatly increases their digestibility. It was of the essence, particularly during dry seasons. A broader selection of dietary energy sources was necessary to fuel the larger brain half a million years ago. A striking increase in human brain size is also one of the major developments in Homo. It has risen from an average ca 600 to 1300 cc in the course of the Pleistocene. As a larger brain is costly in energy, it needs explanation. The social brain hypothesis aims to explain the phenomenon in terms of increased group size and pressures toward social cognition. High-quality diets have been necessary for fueling the larger brain from early times, especially half a million years ago.

The fire was certainly of enormous significance to their lives. It gave them warmth and light, extending their geographical habitat to the colder latitudes as well as into dark environments such as caves. It was inserted in the mythologies of later societies – the Greeks created the story of Prometheus, the great benefactor of humankind, stealing fire from the gods.

Since we carry the memories of our ancestors and all human beings in our subconscious, the fire must take up a great space as a major discovery. The way that humans acquired fire was enshrined in stories. Without fire, humans would not survive very long. Prometheus felt sorry for the human species. The invention of fire was important for many things - like heat, cooking, and hundreds of others. Prometheus stole a lightning bolt from Zeus and gave it to humankind. That is when man discovered fire and was punished for it.

Zeus punished Prometheus. He was chained to a rock in the Caucasus Mountains, and every day an eagle came and ate part of his liver. Each night, his liver would regrow, which meant he had to endure his punishment for eternity. The myth of Prometheus has inspired artists and scientists; in medicine, it has become the symbol of the regenerative capacity of the liver. Live regeneration capacity also shows us that the body may restore itself. Fire has played a major role in transforming the human diet, and apart from its major impact on the environment, it has become socially embedded, even to the point of having religious significance and being incorporated into rituals.

The cooking hypothesis proved that all modern humans need cooked food. Cooking also generally improves the taste and aroma of food, making it enjoyable to eat and easier to digest and changing the nutritional content. Raw foods are more nutritious than cooked foods. Cooked food might be toxic if it is not prepared accordingly.

Interestingly, some vitamins are lost when food is cooked, while others become more available for your body. Some nutrients are easily deactivated or can leach out of food during cooking. Water-soluble vitamins, such as C and B vitamins, are particularly susceptible to being lost during cooking.

Some claim that eating primarily raw foods is the path to better health. The raw food diet comprises mostly or entirely raw and unprocessed foods. A food is considered raw if it has never been heated over 104–118°F (40–48°C). It should also not be refined, pasteurized, treated with pesticides, or processed in any way.

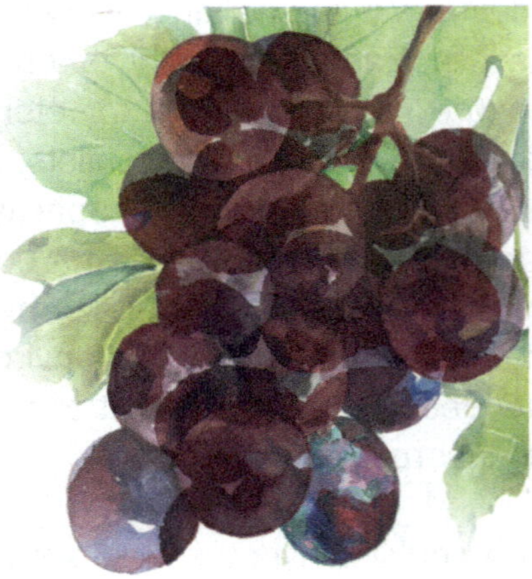

*Figure 8: Grapes have a special place in human evolution. Now it is attracting the attention of science with bioactive molecules and useful phytochemicals.*

Cooked vegetables are higher contents of fat-soluble vitamins than their fresh counterparts. Lycopene is the main carotenoid in tomatoes, and it has been hypothesized to be responsible for reducing the risk of some cancers and heart disease. Cooking tomatoes with olive oil is a characteristic combination of the Southern Mediterranean diet. Previous studies have shown that lycopene absorption is greater from processed tomatoes than from fresh tomatoes since the processing breaks down the tomato cell matrix and makes the lycopene more available. However, it has less vitamin C content compared to uncooked tomatoes.

The possibility that cooking is obligatory is supported by calculations suggesting that a raw food diet could not supply sufficient calories for a normal hunter-gatherer lifestyle. Suppose cooking is indeed obligatory for humans but not for other apes. In that case, this means that human biology must have adapted to ingesting cooked food in ways that no longer allow efficient processing of raw foods.

Since dietary adaptations are central to understanding species evolution, cooking appears to have been a key feature of the environment of human evolutionary adaptedness. Further investigation is therefore needed into how human digestive physiology is constrained by the need for food of relatively high caloric density compared to other great apes.

I operated on a stage 2 lipoedema patient who had no co-morbidities. Her operation was quite difficult. The difficulty in fat aspiration and often clogging of the aspiration tube showed that her lipoedema was deeply inflammatory and fibrotic. I told her, “There should be something wrong with your diet, lifestyle, or hormones.” She told me she followed a healthy, balanced diet. During her postoperative control, she told me she had been drinking liters of milk, particularly Jersey milk. Cow’s milk is a good source of protein, calcium, and vitamin D. However, cow’s milk is also one of the most common food allergens and, as such, is a frequent etiological or triggering factor in a wide range of illnesses. In addition, cow's milk consumption may play a role in the pathogenesis of type 1 diabetes. Allergy is one of the hidden reasons for edema in lipoedema patients. During an allergic reaction, some of the fluid that is part of the blood plasma leaks through the allergically enlarged pores of the temporarily malfunctioning capillaries into the surrounding tissue, causing it to puff up with fluid.

The Paleolithic diet is characterized by lower fat and lower saturated fat intake than Western diets; a balanced intake of omega-6 and omega-3 essential fatty acids; small amounts of trans fatty acids, contributing less than 2% of dietary energy; more green leafy vegetables and fruits providing higher levels of vitamins and other antioxidants. Western diets are characterized by high omega-6 and low omega-3 fatty acid intake, whereas during the Paleolithic period, there was a balance between omega-6 and omega-3 fatty acids. Anthropological researchers have studied diets throughout history and suggest that our hunter-gatherer ancestors consumed omega-6 and omega-3 fats in a ratio of 1:1. The typical diet of modern people has sixteen times the omega-6 than omega-3. Sunflower, corn, soybean, and cottonseed oils contain the highest amounts of omega-6. Olive oil is relatively low in omega 6. Polyphenol-rich extra-virgin olive oil also provides anti-inflammatory and microbiota-modulation effects.

Both ancient and modern hunter-gatherers were free of contemporary inflammatory diseases, like heart disease, cancer, and diabetes, that are the primary causes of death and morbidity today.

Omega-6s and omega-3s do not have the same effects. Scientists believe omega-6s are pro-inflammatory, while omega-3s are anti-inflammatory. A diet with a lot of omega-6 and not much omega-3 will increase inflammation. A diet of a lot of omega-3 and not much omega-6 will reduce inflammation.

However, it is important to ensure your supplement contains enough eicosapentaenoic acid (EPA) and docosahexaenoic acid (DHA). These are the most useful types of omega-3 fats, and they are found in fatty fish and algae.

You can also get omega-3 from nuts, flax seeds, pumpkin seeds, flax seeds, chia seeds, and walnuts. These foods contain alpha-linolenic acid, a small part of which can be converted into EPA and DHA in your body.

The lipoedema diet must be anti-inflammatory. Plant-based diets, including anti-inflammatory herbal plants, are associated with diverse gut microbiota, producing metabolites that have anti-inflammatory functions. The most important aspect of an anti-inflammatory diet is the stabilization of insulin and reduced intake of omega-6 fatty acids. Gluten and other foods which might produce intolerances are eliminated from the diet. My new eating habits and maintenance treatment must be followed for six months to avoid suffering from the "rebound effect."

Lipoedema patients should consume fat which is liquid at room temperature. Such fats are called unsaturated. It's partly true. It's found in vegetable oils, fish, and nuts. In other words, unsaturated fat is an important component of their diet. They improve insulin sensitivity. However, these fatty acids are different than most other fats. They are not simply used for energy or storage; they are biologically active and have important roles in blood clotting and inflammation.

Your body does not have the enzymes to produce them, so you must get them from your diet. If you do not get any from your diet, you develop a deficiency and become sick. That is why they are termed "essential" fatty acids.

Fish and shellfish are great sources of lean protein; many types are rich in heart-healthy omega-3 fatty acids. However, some fish contain worrisome amounts of methylmercury, a toxin especially dangerous to developing brains. That's why women who are or could become pregnant and young children shouldn't eat high-mercury fish such as swordfish, king mackerel, and tilefish. A new study hints that overeating—or the wrong kind—of salmon and tuna can also boost mercury levels. Eating lots of these fish might do more harm than good.

Nuts are rich in nutrients. Brazil nuts contain a huge amount of selenium. Approximately 200 mcg of selenium in each nut. Selenium has anti-inflammatory effects on multiple levels of the inflammatory cascade (Micke et al.). Edema was significantly decreased in two placebo-controlled trials for people with lymphedema after selenium intake.

Nuts may also be a major source of aflatoxin, a potent liver carcinogen whose risk/benefit balance is unknown. Increased nut consumption, as part of a varied healthy diet, is warranted even when aflatoxin exposure is considered.

Our ancestors were not vegetarians. It is not necessary to consume animal foods to maintain good health. In fact, compared with omnivores, vegetarians have a lower risk of developing a number of chronic diseases. However, vegetarians must carefully plan their diet so as not to develop nutritional deficiencies. A balanced, whole-food diet provides essential nutrients for life and good health, including protein, carbohydrates, fat, vitamins, and minerals.

In addition, whole foods contain fiber and a wide range of phytochemicals that may have health benefits. Compared with omnivores, vegetarians have a lower incidence of some chronic diseases. Vegetarian diets also contain lower amounts of pesticides and other toxic chemicals than omnivorous diets since these chemicals tend to bioaccumulate in animal tissues. However, vegetarian diets may be low in a number of micronutrients, including vitamin B12, iron, vitamin D, zinc, iodine, riboflavin, calcium, and selenium. In addition, the protein in most plant foods is incomplete because it contains insufficient amounts of one or more essential amino acids. Failure to provide adequate amounts of any of the eight essential amino acids limits the degree to which dietary protein can be utilized. Proper food combinations can overcome this limitation. For example, grains are relatively deficient in lysine but contain abundant amounts of methionine, whereas beans are relatively deficient in methionine but contain abundant amounts of lysine. When grains and beans are eaten together, these foods complement each other to form proteins of similar biological value to animal protein. Beans and other legumes have been reported to boost blood glucose control and lower serum cholesterol levels.

Hidden food allergy is one of the most common causes of various symptoms and conditions in general medical practice. According to one estimate, as much as 60% of the population suffers from undetected food allergies. In many cases, the successful resolution of chronic health problems that have failed to respond to conventional therapy depends largely on identifying and avoiding allergenic foods.

In my country, soy products are not in our food tradition. Soy is a highly prevalent allergen on the negative side. Furthermore, some practitioners have found that refined soy can be difficult to digest, leading to different gastrointestinal symptoms. It has been shown that soy products (particularly isolated soy protein) inhibit iron absorption, and soy appears to inhibit levothyroxine absorption as well.

Plant polyphenols like isoflavones can be 'bioactivated' by gut microbes to form phytoestrogens which can bind to estrogen receptors. Polyphenol consumption is associated with protection against metabolic syndrome. The capacity of the gut microbiota to bioactivate dietary polyphenols varies considerably between individuals.

When lipoedema and obesity are present together, they worsen one another. First, obesity should be treated, particularly before the surgery. Although calorie restriction can cause weight loss with obesity, it is also helpful in the trunk for lipoedema. Weight-loss programs rely on the maintenance of effortful monitoring of food intake and vigilance of goal processes. Average weight loss typically slows over time because adherence to dietary restriction gradually wanes into a program, and weight regain after successful loss is quite often.

From my experience, I can say that there are higher lipoedema rates in Turkish migrant groups in Germany compared with those living in their original country of birth. It is probably due to diet and lifestyle behavior change and urbanization. They tend to eat a lot of fast food, which triggers lipoedema or speeds up its progression.

Zonulin is considered a biomarker of increased intestinal permeability, and elevated levels have been found in celiac disease. On the other hand, higher zonulin levels are associated with higher waist circumference, diastolic blood pressure, fasting glucose levels, and increased risk of overweight, obesity, and hyperlipidemia. Recent studies indicate that besides digestion and absorption of nutrients and water and electrolytes homeostasis, another key function of the intestine is to regulate the trafficking of environmental antigens across the host mucosal barrier. Intestinal tight junctions create gradients for the optimal absorption and transport of nutrients and control the balance between tolerance and immunity to non-self-antigens.

Exposure to intermittent periods of food shortage sets off a system that prepares for a coming famine by increasing appetite and basal weight above the starting point. Dieting activates the same system, so weight can rebound to above what it was when the diet began. When young people try to lose weight by using willpower to limit their food intake drastically, their regulation mechanisms react with an adaptive response: they often gorge themselves. People who have inherited these genes deposit fat in preparation for a famine that never comes, and the result is widespread obesity (Speakman).

Evolutionary adaptation cannot fix such problems in a short period. Still, it will take hundreds or thousands of generations to solve it, or modern medicine will find a way of speeding up the evolution ( Tooby and Cosmides; Nesse and Williams).

Sharma et al. showed that most types of fruit have anti-obesity effects. It seems to be paradoxical. The incorporation of fruit in the diet drives the gut ecology toward an anti-obese condition by increasing the prevalence of lean-type bacteria but reducing that of obese-type bacteria.

The balance between caloric intake and activity is the basic rule; however, it does not suffice by itself. Stress levels, hormone balance, sleep disturbances, and chemical addiction should be considered and handled thoroughly.

Consumption of a meal with a high glycemic load causes an increase in food cravings, lower energy expenditure, and predisposes to weight gain and obesity.

A low-salt diet needs to be followed with lymphedema and lipoedema. Keeping your salt intake low and increasing your potassium-containing vegetables will improve lymph and blood circulation. The addition of manufactured NaCl salt to the food supply and the displacement of traditional potassium-rich foods by foods caused a 400% decline in potassium intake compared to a 400% increase in sodium ingestion (Cordain). The inversion of potassium and sodium concentrations in diets had no evolutionary precedent and now plays an integral role in eliciting and contributing to numerous non-communicable diseases (Cordain et al.); the modern diet has substantially replaced Stone Age amounts of potassium-rich plant foods with energy-dense nutrient-poor foods and with potassium-poor energy-rich plant foods (especially cereal grains). Himalayan salt has a naturally balanced sodium and potassium and might be a good choice when using salt.

A ketogenic diet is contraindicated for people with lipoedema and lymphedema; as referenced earlier, patients suffering from these conditions have compromised lymphatic systems and struggle with exogenous fats, especially long-chain fatty acids.

For people who experience abdominal pain, fatigue, or other discomforts after the meal, the second option is LSD, which stands for "left side down." You can feel more comfortable breathing, and digestion is easy if you do some LSD. This position also supports the valve at the end of the esophagus, which should be closed once the food enters the stomach. You should allow your digestion to work without the stress of tasks, including talking, driving, and reading. This also increases satisfaction which enhances sleep quality and boosts mood. Lying on your left side helps your energy channel open; you will be breathing through your right nostril, and digestion is encouraged.

You must do this in a relaxed way; otherwise, stress will shut down your digestion.

You should avoid lying down on your right side; it causes esophageal acid exposure, pushing up the undigested food along with the gastric juice and irritating the esophagus. Your digestion process is badly affected.

Walking for 30 minutes just after a meal was more effective for weight loss than waiting one hour after eating before walking. It is quite clear that walking suppresses the glucose increase after a meal. Because glucose increases to its maximum 30–60 minutes after a meal, walking must be started before the glucose level reaches a maximum because once insulin is secreted, it will play a role as an obesity hormone (Hijikata).

Repeated hyperglycemia after meals causes hyperinsulinemia and will result in insulin resistance, which is problematic for people because insulin is the obesity hormone. Suppressing hyperglycemia after a meal will suppress insulin hypersecretion, helping to suppress the storage of internal fat and thus preventing obesity from worsening.

The body has numerous buffering and compensatory systems to maintain its pH balance; the combination of an acidic diet along with emotional stress, high toxin exposure, exercise, and aging can all lead to an increased acid load in the body. With aging, there is a gradual loss of renal acid-base regulatory function and a resultant increase in diet-induced metabolic acidosis while on the modern diet. This acidic load can be more than the body can cope with, and your body faces the challenge of correcting this; otherwise, inflammation and cell damage occur. The prehistoric hunter-gatherer diet was rich in nutrients and low in acid-forming foods; even today, it is still the best diet for human physiology.

Diet diversity or consuming a wide variety of foods will ensure an adequate intake of essential nutrients, leading to better diet quality. Lipoedema patients often ask me if they can drink coffee. Caffeine in coffee makes you feel alert and awake but also leads to a heightened stress response in the body. If you are sensitive to caffeine, try to reduce caffeine consumption by the early afternoon to avoid sleeping problems. Turkish coffee was found to have the highest antioxidant activity among the other types of coffee infusions. With its bioactive polyphenolic constituents, tea also possesses significant antioxidative and anti-inflammatory effects.

Bromelain is present abundantly in pineapple. Various in vivo and in vitro studies have shown they are anti-edematous and anti-inflammatory.

Turmeric, a spice that has long been recognized for its medicinal properties, has received interest from both the medical/scientific world and culinary enthusiasts, as it is the major source of polyphenol curcumin. Most of these benefits can be attributed to their antioxidant and anti-inflammatory effects. Ingesting curcumin alone does not lead to the associated health benefits due to its poor bioavailability, which appears primarily due to poor absorption. For example, piperine is the major active component of black pepper and has been shown to increase bioavailability by 2000% when combined in a complex with curcumin.

The Ancient Greek philosopher Epicurus was born in 341 BC on the island of Samos, a few miles off the coast of modern Turkey. He says that the only intrinsically valuable thing is one's own pleasure. Pleasure is the goal of a happy life. It seems as if he points out our brain's reward system and its pleasure hormone, dopamine. Neurotransmitters are chemicals in our brains that help shape our thoughts and behaviors. Dopamine, one of the main neurotransmitters, is produced mainly in the mid-brain and then moves to other areas of the brain, such as the amygdala, which plays a significant role in our emotional development. It also moves to the prefrontal cortex, which is responsible for thinking, feeling, planning, and taking action. When you do something pleasurable, your brain releases dopamine to make you feel good mentally and physically. This commonly happens when we eat our favorite foods. This reward system is what keeps us motivated and helps us achieve our goals. Our brain's reward system is part of that survival system. We experience an urgent need for food when we are hungry. The brain's reward system rewards food because they ensure our survival. The main rewards are food and reproductive rewards, which facilitate the survival of oneself and offspring. Unfortunately, drugs of abuse operate within these reward systems.

Due to an overflow of energy in modern times, humans have inevitably modified many evolutionary-based behavior patterns. For example, when the body is threatened by energy depletion, humans consume food for its hedonic properties independent of energy status, revealing that the brain reward system plays an important role in feeding behavior. Obese individuals demonstrate increased activation of reward circuitries in response to palatable food compared with lean controls. In Paleolithic times, reward substances were limited. In contrast, today, modern humans are surrounded by many rewarding stimuli in a nearby environment, which can be addictive and inhibit physical activity.

One of the ways to maintain homeostasis is sufficient hydration. It is quite stressful to focus on how many glasses you drink. Observe your urine color. If it is light yellow, you are well-hydrated. If there is no color in your urine at all, likely, you're actually overhydrating. When you overhydrate, you run the risk of electrolyte depletion because you will be urinating too often. It was previously demonstrated that drinking water significantly elevates resting energy expenditure in adults and that low water intake is associated with obesity and lesser success in weight reduction. Water drinking may serve as an adjunctive treatment in patients with impaired orthostatic tolerance. We ignore the quality of water we consume, which is certainly so different from the hunter-gatherers.

# MINDFULNESS

One of the most known definitions for mindfulness is moment-to-moment awareness, cultivated by paying attention in a specific way, in the present moment, as non-reactively, non-judgmentally, and open-heartedly as possible (Kabat-Zinn). It involves slowing down our minds and deliberately grounding ourselves by focusing on what we are experiencing right now (Figure 9).

We are naturally mindful. It is almost certain that our ancestors practiced mindfulness. If they had not been mindful, they would not have survived. We are constantly distracted in today's world. Our minds wander approximately 47% of the time, which directly causes unhappiness (Killingsworth). We dwell on the past, worry about the future, and are distracted by technology.

Fire and conversation are two things that have been of crucial importance for our evolutionary story. Our ancestors ended the day around the campfire, where stories were exchanged. Obviously, this helped them shape their culture, hold the community together, and cooperate with each other. In relation to mindfulness, storytelling involves being present with yourself and the audience.

Although we have been disconnected from our roots in many ways, we still carry the remnants of caveman mentality like herd instinct. Most people act largely emotionally rather than rationally. They follow other people blindly without question. In small-scale environments where we knew others, we evolved. We feel lonely in big cities, surrounded by so many strangers. It is not something that our minds evolved to deal with. The tribal character of the affective link between football fans and their teams is a well-recognized phenomenon. Football fans are passionate, almost tribal in their support and belief in their club.

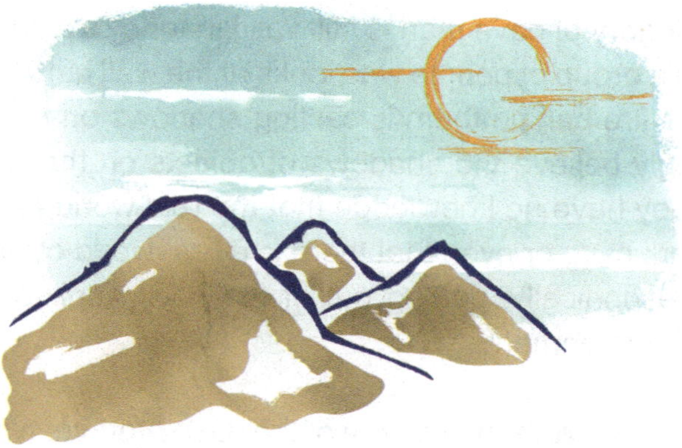

*Figure 9: The mountains, with their difficult living conditions, seem to have provided the continuation of those who managed to survive in human evolution.*

I saw an advertisement. A dentist was explaining the reason for tooth decay to the viewers. Germs decay your teeth, cause mouth odor, and acid attacks your teeth. Combat acid attack on teeth; use this toothpaste to protect your children from that. He was playing on our tribal emotions. We, humans, tend to pay attention to danger.

Awareness of dangers has been important for survival throughout our evolution. We are still tribal.

The allegory of cave man is still valid in today's world. Socrates describes a group of people who looks at the wall before them. The light of the fire behind them is casting shadows on the wall. They misleadingly believe the shadows of objects on the wall are real things. They have no knowledge that the real world exists outside of their dark cave or even that there is a real-world other than their own. Philosophically, getting out of the cave implies reaching a state of enlightenment.

Mindfulness will bring you out of the cave. Various types of brain stimulation by psychological mechanisms, such as mindfulness, are hypothesized to be accompanied by the release of oxytocin in the body.

Oxytocin is an amazing molecule. It is a small peptide synthesized in the hypothalamus of mammal brains. It is made of only nine amino acids and is fragile. Oxytocin is classically associated with uterine contractions and milk letdown for nursing. Oxytocin is a neuropeptide involved in the homeostasis of food consumption and energy.

The brain chemical oxytocin also induces an emotional sense of safety and high levels of social sensitivity. Finally, oxytocin has antioxidant and anti-inflammatory effects, helping to explain the pervasive adaptive consequences of social behavior for emotional and physical health.

Oxytocin appears to make people feel full and reduce overeating. It affects hedonic eating. Several studies have demonstrated the effect of oxytocin's increasing energy intake, decreased food consumption, and contributed to weight loss. Oxytocin's effects on food intake and metabolism suggest its therapeutic potential for treating obesity and binge eating (Hong et al.).

Mindful eating is an approach to food that focuses on individuals' sensual awareness and their experience of the food. It has been recognized that, without behavior change, a diet is useless in the long term. They are all effective in the short term. Conventional weight-loss programs that induce a calorie deficit mostly fail in long-term weight reduction, and none is effective in the long term. The practice of mindfulness has helped thousands of people to live more intentionally and develop the skills necessary to manage chronic diseases, depression, sleeping problems, and anxiety. Mindful eating helps with an eating problem. You can give your body a chance to catch up to your brain and hear the signals to eat the right amount. If you slow down, you can let your mind and body communicate what you really need for nutrition.

I came across a local grocery store which was run by an old man. I wanted him to weigh a kilogram of walnuts. Before weighing it, he told me, "No hurry." He put two walnuts in his old, callous hand and easily crushed them. He offered me a piece of walnut separated from its shell. He said, "First taste it."

I talked to myself by mumbling, "No hurry." I was pressed for time. Why on earth would he not weigh my walnut quickly? He overheard me. He offered me a strawberry by saying the same thing. He said, laughing, "No hurry." People sometimes pass through our lives just to teach us something valuable. Although the phrase "no hurry" is an overused platitude word, his warning stuck in my mind.

Too often, we eat what our brains tell us rather than our bodies. True mindful eating is actually listening deeply to our body's signals for hunger. Put away other distractions and pay attention to your food. Savor each bite. After each bite, check in with your body to see how you feel. Ask yourself if you have had enough.

Our patients are familiar with a ubiquitous cultural figure, Nasreddin, whose anecdotes have an outstanding cultural impact. His story “Taste the Same” gives allusions to mindful eating.

Some neighborhood children see Nasreddin coming from the vineyard with two baskets full of grapes loaded on his donkey. They gather around him and ask him to give them some. Nasreddin picks up a bunch of grapes and gives each child a grape.

“You have so much, but you gave us so little,” the children whined.

“There is no difference whether you have a basketful or a small piece. They all taste the same,” Nasreddin answered.

In our culture, a well-known piece of advice is to chew your food 40 times before swallowing it. This is closely related to mindful eating focusing on what you eat and sensual awareness of the food. It fosters enjoyment and focused tasting of foods. Digestion begins in the mouth. The enzyme amylase, expressed in both the saliva and pancreas, is responsible for starch hydrolysis. Chewing food also stimulates saliva production, which contains amylase (a digestive enzyme), substances that protect the gastric and esophageal mucosa, and compounds that help prevent tooth decay. There is truth in Fletcher’s statement that “Nature will castigate those who don’t masticate.”

It is well known that slow-spaced eating is associated with improved satiety and gut hormone responses, but it might also have some other benefits. For instance, sometimes grains or nuts can smell moldy due to fungal contamination, easily detected by a mindful mind.

# AN ANCIENT HORMONE: VITAMIN D

Vitamin D is an ancient hormone. Plants and animals have produced it from the early life forms of the phytoplankton 750 million years ago to present-day mammals. Its evolutionary past shows why it is crucial in human metabolism. Contrary to its name, vitamin D is not an actual vitamin but a hormone. Vitamin D has the chemical structure of a steroid hormone produced by the kidneys.

The first reference to the physiological effect of sunlight on vitamin D was illustrated by the Greek historian Herodotus. He visited the battlefield where the Battle of Pelusium took place. It was the first major battle between the Persians and the Egyptians. He inspected the skulls of the combatants. He noted that the skulls of the Egyptians were distinguishable from those of the Persians by their superior hardness, a fact confirmed, he said, by the mummies, and which he ascribed to the Egyptians' shaving their heads from infancy, and to the Persians covering them up with folds of cloth or linen. He noted that the Persian skulls were so fragile that they broke even when struck with a pebble, whereas those of the Egyptians were strong and could scarcely be broken even when struck with a stone. Herodotus explained that the Egyptians went bareheaded from childhood, exposing their heads to sunlight. In contrast, Persians covered their heads with turbans shading them from the sun, resulting in skull bone weakness.

Vitamin D is unique because it can be made in the skin from exposure to sunlight. It exists in two forms. Vitamin D2 is found naturally in sun-exposed mushrooms. UVB light from the sun strikes the skin, and humans synthesize vitamin D3, which is the most "natural" form. We do not make vitamin D2. Vitamin D (D represents D2, D3, or both) that is ingested is incorporated into chylomicrons, which are absorbed into the lymphatic system and enter the venous blood. Vitamin D that comes from the skin or diet is biologically inert and requires its first hydroxylation in the liver. This hydroxylation form requires further hydroxylation in the kidneys to form the biologically active form of vitamin D.

Vitamin D provided by plant sources is in the form of vitamin D2, whereas that provided by animal sources is in the form of vitamin D3. These two forms have equivalent biologic potencies. At the same time, vitamin D3 has been shown to be more effective at increasing 25-(OH)D levels.

This vitamin is another evolutionary determinant of our health since it enhances our ability to absorb calcium, iron, magnesium, phosphate, and zinc. Unfortunately, few foods contain vitamin D; thus, direct exposure to sunlight is the natural way to obtain this crucial benefit. Unfortunately, very few food sources naturally contain vitamin D, and the general population, as a result, fails to meet the requirements. Fish have the highest natural content of vitamin D. Other dietary sources are mushrooms, cheese, beef liver and eggs, dark chocolate, milk, and yogurt.

Since an adequate vitamin D intake is hard to achieve through diet alone, dietary vitamin D supplements are usually recommended.

Direct exposure to sunlight is the natural way to obtain this crucial benefit. When an adult is exposed to one minimal erythemal dose of UV radiation (a slight pinkness to the skin 24 h after exposure), the amount of vitamin D produced is equivalent to ingesting between 10,000 and 25,000 IU (Figure 10).

Regarding the amount of vitamin D production in human skin, it depends on several variables, including environmental factors such as geographic latitude, season, time of day, weather conditions (cloudiness), amount of air pollution, and surface reflection, which can all interfere with the amount of UVB radiation reaching the skin. Personal variations represent another group of influential factors affecting vitamin D production in the skin, including age, as elderly people have thinner skin and consequently are less capable of synthesizing vitamin D. Light skin produces up to six-fold the amount of vitamin D produced by dark skin. Skin type, skin thickness, clothing habits, lifestyle, workplace (e.g., indoor versus outdoor), and sun avoidance practices strongly impact vitamin D synthesis. Sunblocks are known to block UVB radiation effectively. Vitamin D3 is synthesized in the skin by a photochemical conversion of provitamin D3 but the necessary rays are only emitted all year round in places below a 35° latitude.

Vitamin D insufficiency affects almost 50% of the population worldwide. This pandemic of hypovitaminosis D can mainly be attributed to lifestyle (for example, reduced outdoor activities) and environmental (for example, air pollution) factors that reduce exposure to sunlight. Wearing sunscreen with a sun protection factor of 30 reduces vitamin D synthesis in the skin by more than 95%.

Vitamin D deficiency often occurs in lipoedema patients. They avoid sun exposure because of psychosocial pressure and fear of edema, which worsens in the hot climate. Because of the unbalanced and Vitamin D-deficient diets, they follow their exogenous intake is limited. In some of them, the requirement increases due to the excess fatty tissue. Adiposity is negatively associated with vitamin D status, and overweight people require 2–3 times more vitamin D than other people to normalize circulating 25-(OH)D levels, which is a very stable vitamin D metabolite.

Nutritional supplementation is not required in humans who have adequate sun exposure. The elderly, the institutionalized, and those living in northern climates likely obtain most of their vitamin D from dietary sources. However, with increasing avoidance of sun exposure by the general population, ensuring adequate dietary intake of vitamin D has become important for the population at large. The major dietary sources of vitamin D are fortified dairy products, although the lack of monitoring of this supplementation results in marked variation in the amount of vitamin D provided.

*Figure 10: You cannot look directly at the sun, only beneficial elements are involved in human evolution.*

Nature probably intended that most vitamin D would be generated by photosynthesis in the skin, with a minor contribution from food sources. However, exposure to sunlight also increases the risk of dermal photodamage and several skin cancers, including melanoma. This was not a problem during human evolution, but with increasing life expectancy, the benefits of UV light for the photosynthesis of vitamin D should be compared with the lifetime risk of skin damage, especially since vitamin D supplementation can safely replace skin synthesis.

The major function of vitamin D is the maintenance of calcium homeostasis. Still, vitamin D insufficiency has also been linked to an increased risk of various diseases, such as autoimmune diseases, diabetes, and cancer. Therefore, there is a growing awareness of vitamin D as a requirement for optimal health. Vitamin D is reported to have anti-inflammatory properties.

Early humans were the naked ape living in the tropics, exposed to high levels of ultraviolet light and vitamin D nutrition, averaging 115 nmol/L compared to today's population averages, which are well below 70 nmol/L. The epidemiological evidence consistently relates lower 25(OH)D to higher disease risk (Vieth).

Vitamin D Insufficiency is usually determined when the total volume of vitamin D (D2, D3) in our blood is less than 30 ng/mL. Vitamin D Deficiency is determined when the total volume of vitamin D (D2, D3) drops further at levels less than 20 ng/mL. Vitamin D Deficiency can contribute to autoimmune thyroid disease. Nutrient deficiencies are usually the result of limited endogenous production, dietary inadequacy, impaired absorption and use, increased requirement, or increased excretion.

# MAGNESIUM IN HUMAN BIOLOGY

Magnesium is extremely abundant in the human body and is the second most common intracellular cation (potassium being the first). It is necessary for the functioning of over three hundred enzymes in humans, with 90% of total body magnesium being contained in the muscles and bones. Therefore, magnesium homeostasis needs to be tightly regulated, which was developed in millions of years. In paleolithic nutrition, magnesium uptake with the usual diet is much higher than today, 600mg /day. Our homeostatic mechanisms and genome are still the same as with our ancestors in the Stone Age. This means our metabolism is best adapted to a high magnesium intake (Figure 11).

Various studies have shown that at least 300 mg magnesium must be supplemented to establish significantly increased serum magnesium concentrations.

If dietary magnesium intake is insufficient, magnesium supplementation is advisable.

Magnesium is considered widely distributed in foods, although the amount of magnesium in food is influenced by various factors, including the soil and water used to irrigate, fertilizers, conservation, refining, processing, and cooking methods. In general, seeds, legumes, nuts (almonds, cashews, Brazil nuts, and peanuts), some fruits, and cocoa are considered good sources of magnesium.

Nevertheless, acidic, light, and sandy soil is usually deficient in magnesium content. Moreover, agricultural techniques, such as the use of potassium and ammonium at high concentrations in fertilizers, lead to magnesium depletion in food (Romani).

Obesity, metabolic syndrome, and type 2 diabetes mellitus are three interrelated conditions that share a series of pathophysiological mechanisms attributable to "low-grade" systemic inflammation. Magnesium deficiency is frequent in obese subjects and is a highly prevalent condition in patients with diabetes or metabolic syndrome. Magnesium deficiency depletion can, directly and indirectly, promote chronic inflammation by modifying the intestinal microbiota (Lobionda et al.).

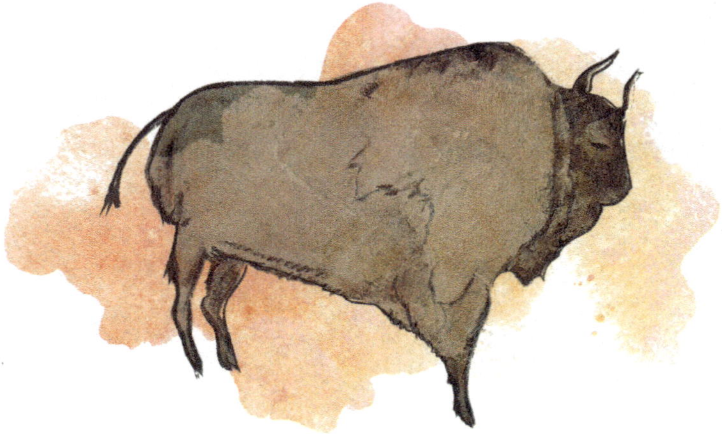

*Figure 11: The theme of hunting and food has an important place in the primitive art made on the cave walls.*

# WE LOST THE ABILITY TO PRODUCE VITAMIN C

Most plants and animals synthesize ascorbic acid for their requirement. The hypothesis is that humans have lost the ability to produce vitamin C for evolutionary reasons. It has been shown that ancestral mammals, living some one hundred million years ago, were actually able to synthesize vitamin C. It contradicts natural selection, highlighting traits that positively contribute to survivability.

It is assumed that humans have included vitamin C-rich foods in their diets for a very long time. The mutation in vitamin C synthesis-related genes has not caused the severe functional deficit, leading to the mutated genotype being passed on to future generations, resulting in permanent loss of vitamin C biosynthesis in humans. Humans subsequently became dependent on dietary vitamin C.

Smokers have long been recognized to have a lower vitamin C status than nonsmokers. This is partly attributed due to the oxidizing properties of tobacco smoke, resulting in an increased turnover of vitamin C. It is recommended that smokers get an additional 35 mg/d of vitamin C. Adequate supplies of vitamin C are necessary for the normal healing process, especially for post-operative patients, because there is rapid utilization of vitamin C for the synthesis of collagen at the site of wound/burns during post-operative period hence.

Normal skin contains high concentrations of vitamin C, which supports important and well-known functions, stimulating collagen synthesis and assisting in antioxidant protection against UV-induced photodamage.

Based on available biochemical, clinical, and epidemiological studies, the current recommended dose for vitamin C is suggested to be 100–120 mg/day to achieve cellular saturation and optimum risk reduction in healthy individuals (Figure 12).

Doctors who are unfamiliar with lipoedema sometimes prescribe diuretics on an empirical basis. In lipoedema, there is no indication for diuretics. They may cause electrolyte imbalance. Furthermore, it might increase pain symptoms. Diuretics should only be used in circumstances of salt and water retention due to cardiac or kidney problems. The development of idiopathic edema in women has been largely attributed to diuretic abuse. Rebound edema on diuretic withdrawal can be an exacerbating factor in many forms of chronic peripheral edema.

Calorie restriction mimetics such as Metformin appear as a convenient way of activating signaling networks associated with the starvation and foraging mode. Herbst suggests that Metformin should be considered early in women with lipoedema Stages 2 and 3, where fibrosis in the fat tissue is prominent, as well as in women who have signs of metabolic syndrome. The same author also suggests that placing lemons, limes, and citrus in water to soak before drinking is a way to intake diosmin throughout the day. Diosmin is a bioflavonoid found in citrus fruits and is traditionally prescribed for treating inflammation associated with chronic venous insufficiency. Women with lipoedema who feel heaviness in their legs, obvious edema, chronic venous insufficiency, or Stages 2 and 3 lipoedema report less pain and improved swelling on diosmin based on the author's experience.

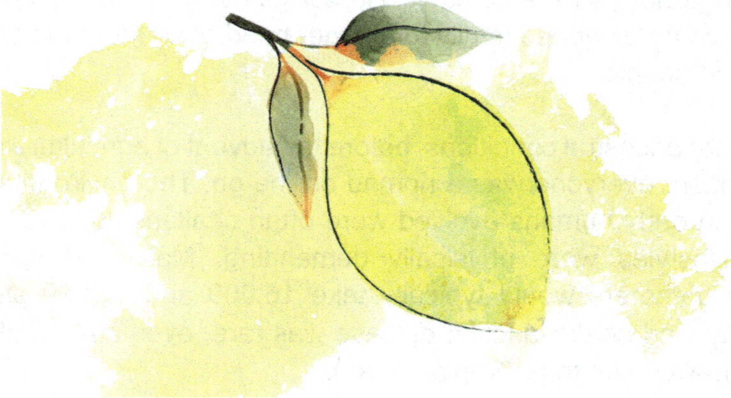

*Figure 12: As we evolved, we lost our ability to synthesize vitamin C.*

# SPONTANEOUS PHYSICAL ACTIVITY

Because hunter-gatherers did not rely on agriculture, they used mobility as a survival strategy. Indeed, the hunter-gatherer lifestyle required access to large areas of land to find the food they needed to survive. This made long-term settlements impractical, and most hunter-gatherers were nomadic. Hunter-gatherer groups ranged in size from an extended family to a larger band of no more than one hundred people.

Under ancestral conditions, before the advent of agriculture and civilization, everyone was a nomad on the go. The environments in which early humans evolved were often challenging, and thus their lifestyles were physically demanding. Male and female hunter-gatherers would typically take 16,000 and 17,000 steps per day, and cardiovascular disease was rare, even among older individuals in the tribe (Kaplan et al.).

Foraging is the vital need to search for food based on locomotion, which requires energy expenditure in the form of running, sneaking, or sprinting to plunder big or small game or climbing and stooping in order to collect honey, berries, nuts, seeds, and plants.

Locomotion, the evolutionary designed solution to dismantle acute stress reactions, is no longer an option in a sedentary working ambiance.

History's greatest minds used the cognitive benefits of moving. Darwin's daily strolls played an important role in the development of his ideas and in reorganizing concepts. He was walking on a sandy path alongside his fox terrier, edged with oaks, many covered with moss. He called it his "thinking path." Aristotle conducted his lectures while walking. Friedrich Beethoven typically worked while walking. One biographer described these short walks as a bee swarming out to collect honey. He would carry a pen and sheets of music paper in case inspiration struck, which it often did. Walking opens up the free flow of ideas.

Because hunter-gatherers did not rely on agriculture, they used mobility as a survival strategy. Indeed, the hunter-gatherer lifestyle required access to large land areas to find the food they needed to survive (Oppezzo M, Schwartz DL).

I saw a stage 2 patient six months after the surgery. She complained of evening edema. I asked her which activities she did during the day. She was sitting all day at work, but she was regularly going to a gym. Her instructor was getting her string jumped for 45 minutes. Her lifestyle was wrong; besides, she was doing the wrong exercises. It did more harm than good. Early occurrence of degenerative changes in the joints and arthroses, especially in the knee (because of wrongly placed stress and excess weight), is quite common in lipoedema patients.

Sedentary life after having worked out 3-4 times a week is not justified. We need to move regularly throughout the day – ideally a little every hour. This movement is often referred to as Spontaneous Physical Activity wherever you are, whenever you can.

Much of our body functions rely on motor activity to keep it working. Our lymphatic system, for instance, needs us to move for its immune and detoxification effects. The lymph system removes body fluids, blood cells, and lipids and serves as a drainage system. The lymph system returns the lymph fluid to the bloodstream, right above the right clavicle. Fluids can easily pool and stagnate when we are not continually moving them against gravity's continually pulling down the action.

Long periods of not-moving can contribute to circulatory issues from this stagnation, from loss of vein integrity, such as edema, cellulitis, varicose veins, hemorrhoids, and diverticulitis.

Our legs have three special "pumps" to aid in circulation: the foot pump, which helps fill the lower leg veins, the thigh pump, which provides general support to the veins and the calf pump, which is responsible for exerting a major "push" on blood in the leg veins, helping it to return to the lungs and heart. In a healthy vein system, each time the calf muscle contracts, or flexes, it forces about 70 percent of the blood in the legs back toward the heart. When the calf muscle relaxes, the deeper veins in the legs are filled with blood. The calf muscles act as a squeezing influence on the deep veins.

The calf muscle pump works best when it is being exercised, which is one of the major reasons why regular walking can play such an important role in maintaining leg circulation and avoiding varicose vein formation in the legs.

At rest, the venous pump is not active. When we go from the seated to the standing position, under the influence of gravity, the weight of the column of blood exerts a pressure of about 80 mm of mercury. After a certain number of steps (about 10 – 25 m), ankle pressure falls to 30 mm of mercury.

The other pump mechanisms are calf pumping, thigh pumping, and diaphragm. The degree of swelling may be related to poor pump mechanics. One of the complaints I often hear from lipoedema patients is edema which sometimes may be persistent even in the postoperative period. Lower extremity fluid pooling is an entity that doctors commonly ignore. It seems that the stimulation of the deep calve muscles (soleus) may improve this situation which may be accomplished via the stimulation of mechanoreceptors on the plantar surface of the feet.

Activation of the calf muscle pump not only reduces venous pressure by increasing venous return but also increases lymph transport.

The plantaris muscle is absent in 7–10% of the human population. It has some weak functionality in moving the knee and gait biomechanics and ankle but is generally considered redundant. The plantaris muscle seems to have a very important proprioceptive role since it has a high density of muscle spindles. The gastrocnemius muscle is prone to painful spasms. The results suggest that plantar vibration serves to significantly enhance peripheral and systemic blood flow, peripheral lymphatic flow, and venous drainage.

During walking, the pump reloads cyclically when the foot is lifted up and empties when weight bearing is applied.

As just described, the plantar venous pump is the only one effective up to the calf, where the calf pump of the soleus muscle takes over its action. Its dual action on both the deep and the superficial saphenous vein circulation underlines the unimpeded blood circulation between the two vascular compartments. In fact, the perforator veins of the foot have an important specific anatomical feature.

Nowadays, a hunter-gatherer group still exists in northeast Tanzania. They spend their days walking eight to twelve kilometers, climbing trees, and digging for root vegetables (Pontzer).

As we have food easily available, permanent and reliable shelter, no predators anymore, and transport to move, this gives us the difficult task of motivating ourselves to get up. The best form of spontaneous physical activity that we can weave into our lives is walking as transport.

Walking is the most natural activity and the only sustained dynamic aerobic exercise that is common to everyone. No special skills or equipment are required. Walking confers the multifarious benefits of this with minimal adverse effects.

Physical activity and exercise undertaken in natural settings, such as parks and forests ("green spaces") and rivers, lakes, the coast, and the sea ("so-called blue spaces,") are strongly recommended for health and well-being, especially mental health and psycho-social well-being. Exercising outside on natural surfaces (the ones we evolved with, like grass and dirt) works more muscles and boosts your balance.

Regular physical activity offers protection against and may be useful as a treatment for a wide variety of chronic diseases associated with low-grade inflammation. It is currently understood that exercise can improve symptoms of lipoedema, despite not decreasing fat accumulation, and it is used as a supportive treatment. Recent findings demonstrate that physical activity induces an increase in the systemic levels of a number of cytokines with anti-inflammatory properties, and skeletal muscle has recently been identified as an endocrine organ that produces and releases cytokines (also called myokines). The discovery of contracting the muscle as a cytokine-producing organ creates a new paradigm: Skeletal muscle is an endocrine organ that, during contraction, stimulates the production and release of myokines that may influence metabolism and modify cytokine production in tissue and organs.

# SEA THERAPY

In my country, the old doctors would prescribe sea air for their patients. The sea air has a therapeutic effect on health and well-being, but we should not limit it to fresh sea air or swimming. There is more to it than seems to the eye. Listening to the rhythmic waves of the sea also has health benefits. It is quite inspirational to view the horizon. It helps you adjust your circadian rhythm to watch the sunrise and sunset. You can collect a few pebbles, twigs so on to make art as a reminder of your holiday. Exercise does wonders for your body, much the same as meditation does for your mind, but viewing or making art helps you connect your mind with your body. You can take a sunbath without sunburn. Our ancestors were exposed naturally to a high incidence of sunlight and ultraviolet radiation, and the region they lived in was devoid of air pollution; they usually did not wear clothes and sunscreens of any type for protection from sun exposure. Bosman et al. presented evidence that skin exposure to narrowband UVB light presented an increase in biodiversity in gut microbial. The human lifestyle concerning sunlight exposure should be considered as one force modulating the gut microbiome. It is a novel skin-gut axis that is associated with health and disease.

You should be close to nature like hunter-gatherers. Bird-David describes hunter-gatherers as individuals who view the world as an 'integrated entity,' embedding themselves within their landscapes. To me, one of the ways of aligning with nature is to collect litter that is strewn on the beach or forest. If you walk on the sand, you will have a double benefit. It is an actual aerobic exercise by breathing in the sea air with the richest oxygen. It cannot be comparable to walking on a treadmill in the stuffy air of the gyms. So, hunter-gatherers have to live not only in harmony with themselves but also with their surroundings. This means that no one is allowed to acquire too much of anything – food, possessions, power, as this may upset the balance, not only of the group but also of the environment. If too much is gathered, not enough may be left to enable natural replacement.

Earthing (the direct contact of the human body with the earth) has been shown to reduce acute and chronic inflammation. It also has been shown to produce symptomatic improvement in chronic muscle and joint pain, a reduction in overall stress levels and tensions, a boost in positive moods, an improvement in heart rate variability, and an improvement in the immune response.

Swimming is the ideal sport against lipoedema. Here the muscular activity takes place in a horizontal position so that there is no danger of the threat of edema, which occurs when the body is upright (orthostatic syndrome). Compared to other exercises, swimming does not cause too much pressure on the body; it reduces the stress in the joints, increases a person's physical strength, and reduces body fat. It also treats blood lipids that cause cardiovascular disorders. Swimming exercise regulates the dopaminergic reward system to decrease high-fat diet intake, thereby controlling body weight to prevent obesity. It may improve metabolic syndrome through multiple pathways.

Swimming is one of the oldest and most basic motor skills of a human. Humans probably started to imitate animal movements (dogs) to swim. 10,000-year-old rock paintings revealed that the people swam breaststroke or doggy paddle.

One of my lipoedema patients (one of my lipoedema teachers!) came from the northern part of the Aegean region of Turkey. She told me how the cold sea water did wonders to subside her edema after the surgery. There, the sea taking water from the cold rivers of Ida Mountain has a unique quality. In fact, she mentioned outdoor hydrotherapy in the sea. Aqua lymphatic therapy significantly reduces limb volume in lymphedema. Water pressure promotes lymph drainage and buoyancy reduces the load on the joints of lower limbs, decreasing the risk of future orthopedic complications.

Cold water swimming has a long tradition in northern countries. However, there is a risk of cardiac problems in people who are not accustomed to cold water, either due to the initial neurogenic cold shock response, a progressive decrease in swimming efficiency, or hypothermia.

There is rising evidence that winter swimmers are more resistant to certain illnesses and infections, experiencing them less frequently and more mildly. The incidence of upper respiratory tract infectious diseases is 40% lower in winter swimmers compared to a control group. Furthermore, it has been shown that swimming in cold water has an impact on immune-specific hematology (Figure 13).

She praised the region she lived. There was an unspoiled seaside town, Assos (Behram), with its ancient period name, where Aristotle found the school of philosophy and a breathtaking landscape on Athena's temple, viewing the legendary city of Troy.

You can question the meaning of life as many ancient philosophers did while walking with sticks thinking back on Aristotle and the Peripatetics' habit of walking while lecturing. In chronic conditions such as lipoedema, psychological reactions are often reported. They have variable moods. Regarding how to cope with chronic stress, there are different approaches.

It is certainly easier to float if you are fat. Fat people tend to float better than skinny people, which may be advantageous. Additional fat reduces overall density and increases buoyancy, which reduces friction and, therefore, increases speed.

Overweight people often find it difficult to find physical activities that will help them get in shape and keep them active and healthy. The high body mass makes many movements difficult, and overweight people are much more likely to get injured due to the mass they have to manipulate with their every move.

*Figure 13: Life began in the seas. Therefore, the sea gives life.*

# VAGUS TONE

When hunter-gatherers experience the life-threatening situation of being attacked by a predator, the sympathetic nervous system is triggered to kickstart the neurobiological responses required for enemies to ward off. Stress was necessary for humans to flee from a predator. The word "fight or flight" describes these threatening circumstances.

This "fight or flight" mechanism is built into our nervous systems. If it is triggered at the wrong time, you may experience a panic attack. It includes body changes, such as increased blood sugar, adrenaline production, altered circulation, etc. Hunter-gatherers quickly got back to normal with no adverse impact on their health. Our ancestors weren't exposed to the chronic stressors of today's world. They did not have overloaded schedules, commutes, unrealistic personal expectations due to media exposure, stress-inducing issues through the media, inefficient bureaucracies, and social pressure to climb the ladder of success.

Like all living organisms, humans maintain dynamic homeostasis, constantly challenged by internal and external stressors. The fight or flight response represents the archaic physiologic response to a threat from a danger signal. Danger and stress factors affecting the Paleolithic ancestors were acute within a relatively short timeframe. Dangerous situations were usually solved within minutes, hours, or days.

In general, fighting and fleeing require augmented energetic demand to support locomotor behavior. However, modern danger signals chronically affect humans' immune systems. This persistent low-grade inflammation state is displayed by the mounting epidemic of non-communicable diseases in Western societies.

During the agricultural revolution, the cooperative hunter-gatherer lifestyle rapidly turned into hierarchal agrarian societies. The agricultural revolution was a key element leading to chronic psychological stress. The widespread appearance of many social roles, pressure to maintain or improve social status and infrastructure, and the higher population densities made possible by agrarian society profoundly increased the impact of infectious disease and parasitism on the population, thus inducing further chronic stress.

Our body knows how to handle acute episodes of stress. The released stress hormones help your mind and body deal with the situation. Short bursts of stress may be beneficial, for instance, to get out of bed in the morning or compete in sports.

Chronic psycho-emotional stress factors trigger an archaic stress system (fight or flight mode). Our bodies were not designed to be constantly activated. This chronic alert situation can trigger a cascade of stress hormones, leading to increased blood pressure, endocrine disorders, gonadal dysfunction, and obesity while worsening the clinical status of many preexisting endocrine disorders.

Hold your arms extended horizontally. Your shoulder muscles first resist the pull of gravity on the weight easily. As the lactic acid accumulates, leading to muscle fatigue, it forces your arm to drop. This is a simulation of rumination, which always remind me of the thinker pose of Rodin. Sitting on a rock, leaning forward with his back hunched over, looking downward with his chin resting on one hand, absorbed in thought. "Rumination" is called rumination because the act of repetitive thinking is similar to the regurgitation of cud by "ruminant" animals such as goats, sheep, and cows. Dwelling on something unpleasant will drag you down. It is a well-established risk factor for the onset of major depression and anxiety symptomatology in both adolescents and adults. In traditional Chinese medicine, there is a statement that says, "Overthinking consumes energy." Mental stress leads to an increase in cortisol, inducing increased appetite and food intake. This phenomenon adds to the current epidemic of obesity.

People are overwhelmed by life, which can be terribly complicated. It results in chronic stress, which leads to your mind and body feeling exhausted. Diogenes of Sinope sees a child drinking water from a natural fountain with his palm. Suddenly, he stands up and throws his only belonging, a mug, at the wall, breaking it into small pieces. He says to himself, "I don't need it either." His action is an extreme example of pursuing a minimalistic life which is the primary condition of happiness. More objects and a more complicated life are equivalent to chronic stress.

The storks are respected birds in Anatolian culture. It has the title "Hacı," which is used for the people who made a pilgrimage. It shows us you consistently cannot achieve your goals without struggle; even if you achieve, you will suffer from various chronic illnesses and pay the price. The storks find a warm column of air; they simply glide. Too much struggle is associated with chronic stress. Life must go on with a smooth rhythm like the hunter-gatherers.

One day, Great Nasreddin's stubborn donkey does not want to go in the direction he wants. Someone asks him, "where are you going?" He says, "The place my donkey wants to go." Do not struggle with life. Let it do things for you.

The vagus nerve is a vital part of the parasympathetic nervous system, which "rests and digests." Laughter has beneficial physiological effects that can be quantified beyond simply saying, "This makes you feel good" Rituals, including chants, prayers, and dance, are practical exercises of the vagal pathways in human history. This nerve is the sensory network telling the brain, particularly the digestive tract (stomach and intestines), lungs and heart, spleen, liver, and kidneys, what is happening in our organs.

Levels of stress in most modern industrialized populations are quantitatively or qualitatively different from those in our early evolutionary past. However, psychological stress is necessary for survival. It prepares the body to cope with the crisis. Chronic psychological stress can lead to a wide range of allergic, autoimmune, and other inflammatory-related diseases.

Put simply, the sympathetic nervous system is the "fight or flight" arm of the nervous system, and the parasympathetic is the "rest and digest" or "feed and breed" side. A sympathetic state is a great state of being when we need some manic energy to work out or meet a deadline, but not so much during our day-to-day life. Because the vagus nerve is vital for the gut-brain connection and other connections within the body, if the vagus nerve is not working correctly, there might be a greater risk of conditions including gastrointestinal issues, heart disease, depression, and anxiety.

If a panther were approaching, however, it would be valuable. For our ancestors, the "fight and flight" mechanism fades when the threat disappears. Modern people keep experiencing the panther threat in their dreams or daily lives.

The vagus nerve brings a wide variety of signals to the brain from the digestive system and organs, and vice versa. It has also been identified as the 'wanderer nerve' due to its long path through the human body.

The microbiota, the gut, and the brain communicate through the microbiota-gut-brain axis in a bidirectional way that involves the autonomic nervous system. Because of its role in interoceptive awareness, the vagus nerve can sense the microbiota metabolites and transfer this gut information to the central nervous system, where it is integrated into the central autonomic network and then generates an adapted or inappropriate response. Therefore, it is considered the sixth sense because of its role in interoceptive awareness.

A cholinergic anti-inflammatory pathway has been described through the vagus nerve's fibers which is able to dampen peripheral inflammation and decrease intestinal permeability, thus very probably modulating microbiota composition. Targeting the vagus nerve, for example, through vagus nerve stimulation which has anti-inflammatory properties, would be of interest to restore homeostasis in the microbiota-gut-brain axis.

We can assume that lipoedema patients have low vagal tonality. Chronic inflammation has been associated with low vagal tonality. The jaw is connected to both the trigeminal and the vagus nerves. Reducing jaw tension helps restore vagal tone. Similarly, decompressing your neck is also helpful. A genuine belly laugh where the head is thrown back for more than 3 seconds activates the vagus nerve, modulates the development of leukocyte cytokine and increases immune function for three days, and has an analgesic effect.

I remember a patient over 50 with a family history of lipoedema in its advanced stages. However, the swelling was confined to her ankle. I dug into her history to find a clue preventing the progression. There was nothing specific with her lifestyle. The thing that attracted my attention was her humor-based positive psychology. In other words, she had a high vagal tone.

Here is an example of a positive mindset example from our culture. One day there was news in every corner of the town about Nasreddin's donkey, which he had lost. When his neighbors heard the news, they got sad and decided to go to mullah's house and help him to find his donkey. So, they came to his house and saw that he was happy and thankful to God. They asked him: "Aren't you sad about losing your donkey?" He laughed and said, "I am happier because God helped me that I was not riding it; otherwise, I would have been lost as well."

Diaphragmatic breathing is defined as breathing in slowly and deeply through the nose using the diaphragm with a minimum movement of the chest. Generally, its practitioners inhale and exhale for approximately six seconds, respectively. Unlike blood, the lymphatic system is not pumped by the heart but relies on the diaphragm's movement.

Martarelli et al. showed that diaphragmatic breathing increased antioxidant activity and reduced oxidative stress after exercise in athletes. Diaphragmatic breathing has the potential to be a non-pharmacological treatment for patients with stress disorder as well as chronic respiratory disease. Chang et al. reported that slow breathing with eight breaths/min makes the balance of the parasympathetic nervous activity dominant.

Patients expect us to give them sophisticated recommendations. "The miracle is in the small things of daily life." Diaphragmatic breathing is easy to do but difficult to develop as a habit. It reminds me of the famous Sufi mystic Bayazid Bastami, who spent most of his life in Anatolia. When he was young, he begged God in all his prayers. 'Give me energy so that I can change the whole world.'He was a revolutionary. "When he became more mature, he started praying: 'This seems too much. Life is passing by quickly. Life is going out of my hands; almost half of my life is gone, and I have not changed a single person, and the whole world is too much.' So, he begged God, 'My family will be enough. Let me change my family.' "And when he became old, "he realized that even the family is too much. If he could change himself, that would be enough. He prayed to God, 'Now I have come to the right point. I would like to change myself.' God replied, 'Now there is no time left. This you should have asked in the beginning. Then there was a possibility.'

# MICROBIOTA

Microbiota refers to the microbial communities living in and on the human body. The human gastrointestinal tract harbors more than 100,000 billion microorganisms, much more than the cells of our organism, and a hundred times more genes than our genome. Microbiome refers to the collective genome of all the microbial cells which reside in the human body.

The precise number of bacteria in the human body is a controversial issue, but it is generally agreed that there are at least ten bacterial cells for every human cell (Ley et al.).

This has led authorities in the field to describe humans as "superorganisms" composed of both human and microbial cells. These microbes inhabit various body organs, including the mouth, gut, reproductive organs, and skin. You provide food, shelter, and a safe habitat for the bacteria. In return, they produce nutrients for the body, including short-chain fatty acids.

Gut microbial synthesis of some amino acids like leucine, lysine, and threonine has also been shown. The body's supply of triglycerides, a prominent energy source during critical illness, is tightly linked to the intestinal microbiota (Schwartz and Brunicardi).

Menaquinones are bacterially produced forms of vitamin K produced by the gut microbiota. Vitamin B-12 is synthesized and utilized by bacteria in the human gut microbiome and is required for over a dozen enzymes in bacteria.

They play important roles in various physiological mechanisms of our bodies. The intestinal microbiome has protective, structural, and metabolic functions in the intestinal mucosa. In return, our bodies provide them with the habitat and food necessary for survival. These short-chain fatty acids can feed the cells in the colon, reduce gut inflammation, help absorb calcium from intestinal cells into blood circulation, and help reduce the risk of colorectal cancer.

Our dietary patterns allow shaping the composition and dominance of certain microbial species residing in the gut. Food components have a key impact on the gut microbiota, influencing its composition in terms of richness and diversity. High intake of animal proteins, saturated fat, sugar, and salt could stimulate the growth of pathogenic bacteria, leading to potential alterations of the intestinal barrier.

The simple concept is that microbes in the gut thrive on what is not bioavailable for the human body. In other words, unavailable food components are the actual food for commensal bacteria in the gut. The main food component impacting gut microbiota composition and activity is fiber. Recent studies suggest that exercise can enhance and enrich the number of beneficial microbial species (Bermon et al.). Exercise is able to enrich microflora diversity. Fasting and circadian rhythm have an impact on it.

Nutrition and symbiosis are two essential aspects of this harmony. Disruption of the symbiosis between host and gut microbiota, the so-called dysbiosis, results in immunometabolic disorders. Dysbiosis is an imbalanced microbial state, often instigated by environmental factors such as broad-spectrum antibiotic usage, which kills both pathogenic and resident microbes, and poor dietary habits. Good bacteria are no more able to control bad bacteria in dysbiosis. The concentration and diversity are the most important part of gut microbiota and keep on changing over time. The "increased intestinal permeability" will produce a chronic low-grade inflammation situation. It might trigger the symptoms in women with a genetic susceptibility to lipoedema. A wide range of factors, such as diet, age, sex, life stage, behavior, ethnicity, and diseases, have been considered microbiome determinants.

Twenty-five hundred years ago, when Hippocrates stated that "All disease begins in the gut," this incredible intuition is applicable to lipoedema.

Consumption of a diet containing high saturated fatty acids and high protein content, medications like antibiotics, and air pollution have a similar effect for pesticides or insects that did on the microflora in the soil. Antibiotics disrupt the natural microbiota in a way that these drugs not only kill the harmful bacteria but also may interfere with the disruption of natural microbiota.

Modern lifestyle might trigger disruption of the biological clock with consequences for the host and the microbiota. Several characteristics of the modern lifestyle, such as working shifts, stress, jet lag, and unusual feeding patterns, have been shown to disrupt the biological clock. Even air pollution may disrupt the gut microflora. Air pollution, which is a complex mixture of gases, may get trapped in the food, and we ingest this contaminated food.

Most human diseases affecting Westernized countries are associated with dysbiosis and loss of microbial diversity in the gut microbiota. Loss of microbiota diversity appears as the most constant finding of intestinal dysbiosis.

Profound changes in diet and lifestyle conditions began with the so-called "Neolithic revolution," introducing agriculture and animal husbandry about 10,000 years ago. Agricultural societies obtained a major part of their daily energy from a single cooked cereal grain (Cordain). It has been hypothesized that bacteria specialized in our gut commensal flora underwent an intense transformation during the social and demographic changes that took place with the first Neolithic settlements (Mira et al.). Chronic non-communicable diseases arise from an evolutionary mismatch. The transition to agriculture could also have altered the proportions of microbial species. Sequencing of calcified dental plaque from ancient teeth has shown that changes in carbohydrate intake appear to have altered the balance between ecological niches of the oral microbiota in favor of cariogenic bacteria (Adler et al.). The fossil record shows that our Paleolithic forbears rarely had cavities (Lieberman), as their diets were largely devoid of simple sugars and starches (Richards).

Lactose intolerance might produce dysbiosis (pathological change in microbiota composition), which might increase hyperpermeability even more.

Leaky Gut is caused mainly by a protein called zonulin. There is evidence that gluten causes a large zonulin release. When tight junctions loosen, protein structures go into the bloodstream without being digested. The immune system reacts against them, causing an immune/inflammatory reaction.

There is evidence of a correlation between total bacteria and serum zonulin levels, suggesting that the gut microbiota may cause increased zonulin levels and subsequent abnormal gut permeability to endotoxin, and ultimately, micro-inflammation has been reported in obesity.

Diversity is critical in microbiome health. How to restore the bacterial diversity of the host microbiota?

I came across a farmer on occasion. Her story was really inspiring for understanding the term biodiversity in a macro system. She bought a piece of land that was in poor condition because of previous conventional farming techniques. Conventional farming eliminates biodiversity because of pesticides and herbicides and reliance on monoculture. She let the land fallow for a year and used organic fertilizers to improve soil microbes and feed the soil. She planted heirloom seeds that are resilient to diseases. She used the herbs like thyme and lavender to keep pests away. She said to me, “Earthworms were first seen. Ladybirds, wasps, and spiders later came, and some other beneficial insects came out sequentially as pest controllers." This is biodiversity, or the life variation, essential to healthy ecosystems. Organic agriculture sustains the health of soils and the ecosystem.

This biodiversity in a macrosystem bears a resemblance to one of the bacteria in the microsystem of our guts.

Some patients told me their bowel problems went away after the surgery. I clearly remember two patients diagnosed with autoimmune diseases whose symptoms dramatically decreased. Since the gastrointestinal tract hosts 70% of the immune system, the leaky gut problem might have gotten better. Was it because they followed a healthy diet, was it part of improved metabolism after the surgery, or both?

For modern hunter-gatherers, The Hadza microbiome is markedly different from the microbiomes of people in industrialized countries. Most notably, it boasts more taxonomic diversity and greater stability, which are key markers of microbiome health.

Butyrate-producing gut bacteria could decrease gut permeability by decreasing zonulin levels and lowering inflammation. Walnut consumption affects the composition and function of the human gastrointestinal microbiota, increasing butyrate-producing bacteria.

Our ancestors were exposed to all kinds of microbes in the dirt, and they spent time with animals most days; they did not use antibiotics that destroyed microbes. Our immune systems, which are accustomed to fighting external enemies, do not face the same challenges they once did. This may cause to attack our own cells leading to a war called autoimmunity, which is linked with diabetes type I, arthritis, multiple sclerosis, and maybe even cardiovascular disease.

We undervalue host-microbe and microbe-microbe interactions on the human skin surface, creating a complex and dynamic ecosystem. Their beneficial function is much like that of the microflora of the gut. The skin microbiome is essential to the skin protection and immunity processes that serve as a barrier to certain allergens and contaminants in the setting. In this extremely distinct epidermal microbiota, it has been shown that

Staphylococcus epidermidis and Staphylococcus hominis have an additional protective role for our skin.

They secrete antimicrobial peptides which kill Staphylococcus Aureus, a pathogenic bacterium. Frequent washing has been reported to weaken the skin barrier, resulting in skin irritation and microbiome changes on the skin of the hand. The gut model can be adapted to the skin in the near future, and microbiota in the skin might become a new focus for treating certain diseases.

Fermented foods vary from country to country. In our culture, shalgam juice, hardaliye, boza, pickled olives, pickle, and vinegar, which are obtained from vegetables, fruits, and cereals, are among the popular ones. Koumiss, cheese, soudjouk, tarhana, butter, yogurt, and kefir are the other traditional Turkish fermented foods made of milk.

Prebiotics are a form of dietary fiber that feed the "friendly" bacteria in your gut. For instance, garlic acts as a prebiotic by promoting the growth of beneficial Bifidobacteria in the gut. It also helps prevent disease-promoting bacteria from growing. Apples are delicious fruits with fiber. Pectin, a type of soluble fiber, accounts for much of an apple's total fiber content. The pectin in apples has prebiotic benefits.

Probiotics have been defined as viable microorganisms. Fermented foods are defined as foods or beverages produced through controlled microbial growth. Therefore, they contain potentially probiotic microorganisms, but all fermented foods do not contain probiotics. Some foods, like baking and canning, undergo steps that remove the probiotics, as with beer or wine, or make them inactive.

The surrounding food matrix appears to play an important role in the survival of probiotic strains via its buffering and protective effect against gut conditions (e.g., low pH, bile acids). Fermentation-derived metabolites may exert health benefits. For example, lactic acid bacteria generate bioactive peptides and polyamines, potentially affecting cardiovascular, immune, and metabolic health. Fermentation may convert certain compounds to biologically active metabolites. Lactic acid bacteria can convert phenolic compounds (flavonoids) into biologically active metabolites. Food components found in fermented foods, such as prebiotics and vitamins, may also exert health benefits.

Kefir is the fermented food most commonly investigated in terms of its impact on gastrointestinal health. Observational and interventional studies in humans suggest that the consumption of fermented foods is associated with protection from metabolic and immune-mediated diseases. They can be an effective vector for the delivery of probiotics to the gut because of their nutritional value and acidic nature.

Prebiotics are considered food for bacteria. Naturally, prebiotics are found in foods rich in fiber, like vegetables, fruits, whole grains, and legumes such as peas and beans. Bacteria can convert nondigestible food components like fibers that fail to be broken down by the host digestive enzymes. The word prebiotics might be summed up as being fiber. They are nondigestible carbohydrates that act as food for probiotics.

Certain foods are approached with a particular interest and are even considered future medicines. These special foods have been defined as "adaptogens," of which garlic is a prime example (Adelman and Haushofer). Hippocrates referred to these special foods more than 2300 years ago, saying, "Let your food be your medicine."

# CIRCADIAN SYSTEM

Homeostasis is the ability to maintain internal stability in an organism in response to environmental changes. In homeostasis, the system continuously changes the pH of blood acid, blood pressure, blood sugar, electrolytes, hormones, and temperature to have the body to survive and function correctly.

Yogurt happens after a set of chemical reactions. Lactose in milk is fermented by Lactobacillus into lactic acid, causing the proteins in milk to coagulate. Billions of such chemical reactions happen inside our body and the interstitial fluid that surrounds all cells to maintain homeostasis. The burden of and accompanying bad habits such as smoking, overeating, alcohol, and poor-quality sleep cause an allostatic overload. Although the effects of short-lived stress are reversible, chronic stress may permanently affect our brains.

A central tenet in medicine is that effective therapy must re-establish the disrupted homeostatic mechanisms. In our bodies, a self-regulating process exists that maintains internal stability. If homeostasis is not restored, our body cannot function properly; the imbalance may lead to disease or even death.

Circadian coordination is essential for good physical and mental well-being, which is a critical part of homeostasis. In 1729, French scientist De Mairan noticed that the mimosa plant opened its leaves during the day and closed them at night. He placed the plant overnight in a cupboard. When he opened the cupboard doors the next morning, the plant's leaves were completely unfurled, although it was not exposed to sunlight that day. The scientist concluded that the mimosa must have some sort of built-in biological clock that lets it know what time it is.

Daily changes of all species in their physiology are not simply a response to the 24-hour changes in the physical environment imposed by the earth turning on its axis. Instead, they arise from a timekeeping system within the organism. This timekeeping system, or biological "clock," allows the organism to anticipate and prepare for the changes in the physical environment associated with day and night, thereby ensuring that the organism will "do the right thing" at the right time of the day.

The main conclusion was that the body has an internal clock mainly affected by the sun's light/dark cycle. Your body's circadian clock responds to light as a signal to be awake and dark as a signal to fall asleep. Life forms on our planet have evolved under the influence of a daily light-dark cycle. Daily changes in light and darkness result in diurnal rhythms.

Many body processes have daily fluctuations, including body temperature, blood pressure, and hormone levels. Melatonin peaks late at night and decreases in the morning, whereas the hormone cortisol peaks in the morning.

The circadian rhythm initiates the so-called cortisol awakening response independent of hunger, thirst, or other motivational drives.

Cortisol plays a specific role in synchronizing the body. Cortisol levels increase autonomously in the morning before awakening to provide preferentially glucose for the brain and fatty acids for skeletal muscles to support foraging behavior or physical activity in general. In the morning, the circulating amount of glucose rises, a fact known as the dawn phenomenon. Levels of cortisol display a sharp increase immediately upon awakening, known as the cortisol awakening response. This cortisol awakening response is thought to prepare the brain for upcoming challenges. General good health has been linked to a higher cortisol awakening response. In the morning, activities that may help encourage a healthy cortisol awakening response include exposure to bright, natural light immediately on waking, going outside, and performing exercise within 30 to 45 minutes of waking.

Long-term stress has been shown to lower the cortisol awakening response and contribute to morning fatigue, pain, and inflammation. In healthy participants, the cortisol awakening response involves a sharp increase in cortisol secretion following awakening, which peaks between 30 and 45 minutes and returns to baseline at 60 minutes post-awakening. Lower cortisol levels are present at the initial part of sleep, whereas there is an increase at the end of the sleep period, which peaks after waking.

All behavior patterns in the context of physical activity are associated with the energy demands of neurons and skeletal muscles. However, energy intake was never predictable before the era of agriculture.

Exposure to light at night disturbs the rhythm, leading to sleep disturbances.

Other environmental and behavioral time cues, termed "zeitgebers," such as the timing of meals, exercise, and sleep-wake cycles, can "fine-tune" the central clock. Indeed, our prevailing modern lifestyle (round-the-clock access to energy-dense food, low levels of habitual physical activity accompanied by periods of prolonged sitting, and inadequate quality/quantity of sleep) interacts with underlying biology to create an environment in which circadian rhythms are disrupted, often resulting in a plethora of metabolic conditions (Bishehsari et al.).

We need to "live within the life cycle of the ecosystems we occupy." Our ancestors knew the food rhythms of the season. They hunted and trapped year-round.

In addition to light, which is one of the main signals that set our biological clocks, other important factors, such as nutrition, can also affect our biological rhythms. This means that what we eat can change the way our bodies function. For example, when eaten, plants contain substances that serve as signals that regulate our clocks.

It is claimed that some of these plant substances provide our bodies with information about the environmental conditions in which those plants were grown, and these signals allow us to adapt to the various seasons of the year. If we consume fruits and vegetables produced where we live when they are in season, our bodies will be ready to make the changes required to face the upcoming season. Eating more seasonal food is one proposal for moving towards more sustainable consumption patterns, based on the assumption that it could reduce the diet's environmental impact.

Polyphenols are substances produced by plants that are good for our health—they help to prevent several diseases, such as high blood pressure and obesity. In addition, polyphenols can also affect biological rhythms. More than 8,000 different polyphenols are present in fruits, vegetables, cocoa, and beverages such as tea or wine. Plants produce these compounds in response to environmental stresses such as cold temperatures, rainfall, or drought. Therefore, each plant has a specific, unique polyphenol composition depending on the environmental conditions in which it was grown. Those polyphenols provide information about the environment during the plant's growing season.

But today, all fruits and vegetables can be eaten throughout the whole year. For example, the orange, a winter fruit, is grown and harvested during the winter in South Africa and can be eaten in Europe during the spring and summer. According to the xenohormesis theory, Europeans will receive "winter" signals if they eat this orange, and their body will prepare for winter. This can cause a conflict, or desynchronization, between his internal clock and the actual environmental conditions.

Xenohormesis theory proposes that some of these plant substances provide our bodies with information about the environmental conditions in which those plants were grown. These signals allow us to adapt to the various seasons of the year. In other words, if we consume fruits and vegetables produced where we live when they are in season, our bodies will be ready to make the changes required to face the upcoming season. Eating more seasonal food is one proposal for moving towards more sustainable consumption patterns, based on the assumption that it could reduce the diet's environmental impact. Eating the same fruits out-of-season produce different biological responses.

Disruption of the circadian system can alter microbiome communities and perturb host metabolism, energy homeostasis, and inflammatory pathways, leading to metabolic syndrome. We can assume that someone with a disrupted circadian rhythm has dysbiosis. While correcting the circadian rhythm, we should repair and improve the ecology of gut flora.

Disruptions in sleep patterns are associated with increased body fat and altered metabolism, although the cause-effect relationship for these associations has yet to be elucidated.

The sun regulates much of human behavior. Our ancestors stayed awake three to four hours past sunset, with no light exposure other than the faint glow of a small fire that would keep animals away and provide a bit of warmth in the winter. They must have woken up with the first sunlight and looked at it with great admiration. They must have started a new day with a sharp increase in cortisol levels.

The "jet-lag syndrome is typical of the desynchronization of the circadian rhythm. If you experienced it, you would have felt how it destroyed the balance in your body. Because it is an acute situation, we know its impact is quite sharp. Most people, like lipoedema patients, live in a damaged circadian rhythm, but they are unaware because of its chronic nature.

I clearly remember a patient who complained of difficulty in nose breathing during sleep. The nasal passage was clear, with no visible mechanical obstruction. She reported after the leg liposuction, the difficulty was completely restored. It might be attributed that the nocturnal fluid shift improved. Lower extremity fluid pooling has been associated with impaired sleep quality. The fluid accumulating in the lower extremities during the day moves toward the head during sleep. Fluid pressure in the neck may collapse the upper airway, which predisposes individuals to sleep-disordered breathing (Bradley & Floras, Shepard et al.). When I see somebody with mechanical obstruction in the nasal airway, I recommend to have the obstruction corrected. A lipoedema patient with nasal obstruction can never get out of the vicious circle.

We, humans, tend to deprive ourselves of sleep. Let alone a lipoedema patient; a healthy person may be negatively affected by sleep deprivation.

The biological clock tells your body when it's time to perform your everyday necessities and when to be active and inactive over a roughly 24-hour cycle, from sleeping to eating. Your energy levels fluctuate throughout the day. If you notice daily energy peaks and dips, you will be able to function your best daily performance.

It is actually not just one internal clock. At certain times of day and night, and according to internal and external cues, these clocks start predictable biological processes, like hormone production, temperature regulation, blood pressure, and the most well-known of all — your sleep-wake cycle.

In the old stone age, there were no consistent sources of food. Human nutrition used to be subject to weekly, monthly, and seasonal fluctuations. Anyhow, in periods of fasting, humans should have been able to use stored energy, if necessary, for many hours or even days without any food supply. For that reason, in late summer or at the end of a rainy season (the time of plenty), it became extremely important for our Paleolithic ancestors to take advantage of easily digestible carbohydrates, such as ripe fruits, to build up body fat, preparing for a scarcer food supply during winter or dry season (the time of caloric or carbohydrate restriction.). Homo sapiens adapted to these seasonal changes by developing several survival mechanisms. One example is given by the fructose transporter, which enables fruit-derived fructose to be allocated into cells independent of insulin. In contrast to glucose (20%), the liver immediately converts nearly 100% of all ingested fructose into fatty acids and then further esterified to store triacylglycerols. Adipose tissue, responsible for 60% of all triacylglycerol accumulation, can store large amounts of excess free fatty acids. The mechanism to convert fructose into fat was a vital survival advantage for our ancestors, particularly when facing seasonal starvation.

Thus, intermittent fasting and longer-term caloric as well as carbohydrate restriction are parts of our genetic heritage. All three can lower glucose, insulin, triacylglycerol, and lipid accumulation and, at the same time, increase insulin sensitivity while increasing HDL-cholesterol123. Intermittent fasting was proven to significantly reduce low-grade inflammation by degrading IL- 6, TNF-alpha, and CRP. Examples include but are not limited to, periodic fasting or calorie restriction (e.g., once a year as traditionally practiced within the world religions), occasional meal skipping, ketogenic diets (e.g., during the winter months), and a combination of endurance and strength training several times per week (Freese et al.).

Hunter-gatherers foraged for food in order to survive. Our ancestors commonly experienced a fasting period until they found their food. Those early hunter-gatherers were probably used to going a day or two, perhaps longer, with little or nothing to eat. The fasting period serves as a time for standby and repair so that the organism can harvest energy when food becomes available. Neuronal networks in the brain and related critical thinking and decision-making developed as they were hunting and foraging in a fast state in hazardous environments. It was reflected in their artistic expressions in the caves, with food-centric themes depicting game animals or domesticated food animals.

For most of human history, people ate one or two meals daily. The time-restricted eating patterns or one meal-a-day diet mimic this ancient phenomenon.

Results reveal that Intermittent fasting directly influences the gut microbiome in bacterial abundance and metabolic activity by contributing to circadian rhythmicity in the host.

# COMPRESSION SOCKS ARE FRIENDS OF LIPOEDEMA PATIENTS

Compression garments help compensate for the loss of skin elasticity and support tissues. This can decrease pain and enhance muscle pumping action to move fluid out of swollen areas. This helps the body feel less heavy and makes moving and walking easier. It might help prevent lipoedema from progressing by helping lymphatic and vascular circulation. Compression therapy can naturally not reduce adipose tissue mass but can prevent additional edema formation and thus reduce the resulting tension and pain. Compression therapy can help mobilize patients and thus prevent or ameliorate obesity.

If compression is only used on swollen areas closer to the trunk, such as thighs and knees, the uncompressed lower legs and feet are vulnerable to increased swelling. This might worsen an unrecognized lipoedema in the lower legs. It squeezes the fluid out of the limb with force, like squeezing toothpaste out of a tube.

Graduated compression stockings exert the greatest degree of compression at the ankle, and the compression level gradually decreases up the garment. They are often used to treat chronic venous disease and edema. Most notably, graduated compression socks are better for use when gravity is a concern. Graduated socks are usually better if you are going to be sitting or standing for long periods.

The pressure gradient ensures that blood flows upward toward the heart. Graduation compression can reverse venous hypertension, augment the skeletal muscle pump, facilitate the venous return, and improve lymphatic drainage. Although the exact mechanisms remain unclear, it also initiates complex physiologic and biochemical effects involving the venous, arterial, and lymphatic systems. Limb oxygenation increases with the use of graduated compression stockings, especially with high-compression stockings. Levels of proinflammatory cytokines are significantly reduced following compression therapy.

Low compression usually refers to a pressure of less than 20 mm Hg or Class 1; medium compression to a pressure of 20-30 mm Hg or Class 2; and high compression to a pressure greater than or greater than 30 mm Hg or Class 3.

Textured circular knit compression garments have less compression (12-21 mmHg), but the micro-massage created by the weave in the fabric stimulates the superficial lymphatics and compensates for having less pressure. They are also generally more comfortable to wear and easier to put on and take off, but they may not be strong enough to support larger bodies or stage 3 and 4 lipoedema. In those cases, flat knit might be a better compression alternative.

I often asked if they felt much pain after the surgery. My observation is that pain after the surgery is quite tolerable. If a patient says she feels severe pain, I tell her to check her stockings. There should not be any folds in the fabric to allow the pressure across the limb to be uniformly distributed and to avoid having a higher pressure over a specific area. Folds and pleats may exert a strangling effect. Compression stockings require careful application and close supervision to minimize potential risks.

It has been reported that the reduction of edema and pain in the legs during the course of the day can be accomplished with the use of elastic stockings, as well as walking for 50 minutes in the late afternoon while wearing elastic stockings (Carvalho et al.).

Contact dermatitis, skin discoloration, and blistering may develop in patients who are allergic to stocking content.

# LIPOSUCTION AS THE MAIN TREATMENT OF LIPOEDEMA

Liposuction is the most effective solution for lipoedema. Because liposuction removes the inflammatory fat cells permanently, it may slow down or even stop the disease's progression with a suitable postoperative program. Lipoedema may get back to its latent phase. Although it was a safe procedure, clinical studies for legs appeared in the literature in the 90s.

Liposuction of calves and ankles has always been considered a "difficult area," and experienced liposuction surgeons with specific training should only perform it. Interest in the concept of body contouring was lost for a long time following Dujair's case. Fortunately, we can do various aesthetic surgeries safely nowadays with evolving technology.

Suzanne Geoffre was a young Parisian woman, a model, and a professional dancer. She had formerly worked for the Poiret Haute Couture before she had recently founded a prosperous maison de couture in the Concorde district after having saved for a number of years. After the war, skirt lengths continued to rise-ten to twelve inches above the floor, now hemmed at the knee. Her heavy legs were probably due to lipoedema. Her ongoing marriage and the pressure of changing fashion trends stressing a leaner body figure exposing the legs stirred her desire to have slimmer legs. Geoffre consulted with Dr. Leopold Levy, a specialist in sicknesses of circulation and obesity. Levy told her there was no abnormal finding and there was not much he could do for her.

Levy recommended Dr. Dujarrier, and Geoffre went directly to his office. Dujarrier examined her and explained that she had "a simple excess of fat" in her legs, and told her that it would be very easy to remove. The operation took place the next day, 28 February 1926.

Dujarier was a renowned osteoarticular surgeon who was not well-versed in cosmetic surgery. Dujarier agreed to operate free of charge in his department of the Beaujon hospital and not in his clinic, presumably because of the exploratory nature of the procedure and its scientific interest.

The young woman was admitted to the hospital the day after her first consultation with Dujarier, and the operation took place the following day. She was told the surgery would be neither lengthy nor particularly risky. But the procedure proved more complex, and the removed fatty substance was larger than expected.

The operation was a disaster. The concept of removing excess fat from localized body sites to achieve similar gains is credited to Charles Dujarrier, who, in France, attempted to remove subcutaneous fat using a uterine curette on the calves and knees of a ballerina in 1921. He had removed too much tissue, and there was excessive tension in the closure. The surgeon had difficulty suturing and elected not to operate on the second leg. After the surgery, the patient's state quickly deteriorated. Within a few days, gangrene set in, and the surgeon had to amputate the leg. Suture tension was responsible for gangrene that required amputation of the operated leg.

It has been assumed that he used a uterine curette to scrape the fat from the legs, anticipating having to sew up Geoffre's slimmer legs. Dujarier excised more of the outer skin than he should have.

He then tried to bring the wound's edges together and sew them with stitches, but the amount of flesh he had cut out was too great, and the edges would not come together. As a result, Dujarrier had to "tie up this leg… like a sausage." Shortly after that, Geoffre found that she had lost all feeling in her foot and could not move it. On 20 March, Dujarrier told Geoffre that gangrene had developed and that her leg would have to be cut off or she would die within forty-eight hours. Geoffre refused, saying she would rather die. She was finally persuaded to undergo the operation after her fiancé, M. Le Guen, offered to marry her in the hospital. The couple was married that evening, and the next day, the leg was amputated.

The rumor is that Dujarier agreed to perform the surgery mainly to enhance his prestige, as Geoffre's social status could bring him more upscale patients.

Shortly after the catastrophic result, all cosmetic surgery procedures were banned. It was reported that Geoffre's "deformity" did not exist, and there was nothing seriously wrong with her body that would justify a surgeon's operation since beauty ideals were ephemeral (Comiskey). The procedure was performed by a surgeon who is not an aesthetic plastic surgeon, but the specialty of aesthetic surgery was blamed. This unfortunate complication arrested further progress in this field. Modern liposuction began with the technique and instruments of Giorgio Fischer, and his father, Arpad Fischer, in Italy, in 1974.

As to the lessons we take away from that tragedy: Always get the specialist to perform a procedure. Always ask for the previous experience of the surgeon about the operation. Never undergo an operation when you are really pressed for time.

# UNTREATED LIPOEDEMA

When I let the patients tell their stories, they usually focus on the disease's functional, psychological, and social aspects. The onset of symptoms, progression, what triggers the symptoms, and when it flares up allows me to draw the disease progression graphic. Some patients do not want to undergo any surgical treatment because they have some comorbidities that put them at risk, and some delay the surgery because of financial or other reasons. They all want to know what if they do not undergo surgical treatment. It can be deduced from their data and family history, which may illustrate how the long-term results of the disease would affect them. Patients often say, "I do not want to look like my mother or grandmother when I get old." Their life quality is quite poor. "Their mother's and/ or grandmother's situation forces them to undergo surgery.

Lipoedema is a progressive disease. Its course has a worsening feature, resulting in a general decline in function. Although it is difficult to determine the course of lipoedema, its course draws parallelism with their relatives' situation. Untreated lipoedema may result in secondary problems, including osteoarthritis, obesity, reduced mobility, psychological impairment, and lowered self-esteem. The weight of the excessive fat can cause the knees to knock inward and impair the walk. The problems caused by wear and tear of the joints dramatically increase in lipoedema patients. As mentioned, in the later stages, secondary lymphedema may occur due to an imbalance in the amount of fluid produced and drained by the lymphatic system. Lipoedema poses a significant psychosocial burden for most patients, and associated effects often limit exercise capacity.

Disease progression is heterogeneous and highly variable from one individual to the other. Some women's lipoedema stabilizes over time, while others exhibit gradual disease progression with sudden stress-induced exacerbation (i.e., pregnancy or surgery).

Especially in stage 3 of lipoedema, there is a lymphatic flow disorder due to the increasing stenosis of the lymphatic vessels by the sudden growth of the adipose tissue. With the overwhelmed lymph circulation, the ability to clear fatty acids from the affected tissue is compromised, and secondary fat accumulation occurs.

Parts of the infected lymphatic vessels may be destroyed following a soft tissue infection. This blocks the flow of lymph (the fluid in the lymphatic system), causing it to build up. That results in permanent swelling and poorer circulation in the tissue, increasing the risk of developing further bacterial skin infections.

Most of the patients are labeled or misconstrued as obese. Lipoedema is often confused with obesity. Obesity is the accumulation of excess fat stored centrally inside the abdominal cavity or belly. At the same time, lipoedema is the excess accumulation of fat out of proportion on the extremities.

What can make it confusing is that lipoedema and obesity may coexist. Obesity may develop as a secondary condition due to mobility problems caused by lipoedema. Obesity can also complicate lipoedema.

In advanced stages, fibrosis, skin tightening, and subcutaneous cell tissue might produce musculoskeletal alterations and difficulty with walking, leading to disability due to orthopedic complications.

Lymphatic drainage is impaired when lipoedema remains untreated for years and the lymphatic vessels are progressively strained. It has also been demonstrated that multiple micro lymphatic aneurysms at the thigh, ankle region, or foot. Adipocytes are well known to develop dramatically in the presence of lymphatic fluid (Harvey et al.).

The only effective nonsurgical treatment method is the combination of manual lymph drainage and compression treatment. I used to send my patients to the centers for manual lymph drainage. After working with a French lymph therapist, I noticed it has nothing to do with lymph drainage therapy. She came to Istanbul in pursuit of her love. As Tolstoy said, stories start when a foreigner comes to the town or leaves the town. Her contribution to my story was that she made me aware of what real lymph drainage was. The patients had had a kneading massage of their legs or vacuum therapy, which they should avoid before I knew her. Lipomatous tissue is an inflammatory, tender, and damaged one. We should not add extra damage to it.

# MY CAREER JOURNEY IN LIPOEDEMA

Liposuction is the main surgical intervention for lipoedema. I first published an article about the use of liposuction under a tourniquet for the kneecap area in the "Journal of Aesthetic Surgery" in 1998. It was a liposuction technique under a tourniquet which allowed the surgery to be performed conscientiously and safely. It is known that the leg has only one layer of subcutaneous tissue, leaving little margin for error. This peculiarity calls for a different approach than that of the other regions. This approach goes one step further in the process of leg sculpting. It aspirates pure fat with no blood. It is truly selective adipoaspiration. The technique renders easy the appreciation of the final result. What you see at the end of the procedure is the final result. To be honest, I was not familiar with lipoedema at that time. Therefore, I applied the procedure of liposuction only to the places they complained about. It was the kneecap area. I expanded the area I treated to the lower legs and ankles. I used a limited version of the superdry technique, which was actually two-dimensional. It evolved to the superdry 3D by the influence of accumulating experience, which became a circular and extensive technique. The critical point of liposuction was to aspirate fat in a circular way; otherwise, it would definitely recur without an aesthetically pleasing appearance. Using a tourniquet eliminated blood loss even during the preoperative period, which was further improved by the preemptive injection of a mixed solution for the postoperative third space blood loss. I particularly injected the solution alongside the major veins and lymphatic channels.

I used to treat my lipoedema patients from a surgical point of view, using mostly my personal technique, superdry 3D, and its combination of other liposuction techniques. I noticed that it was not sufficient to get the best result. Dynamic aesthetics and the appearance of movement should be taken into consideration. Therefore, I called the technique superdry 4D considering the movement of muscles.

In aesthetic surgery, some procedures are closely related to creating sculptures in terms of three-dimensional forms and composition. But nothing else can compare with lipoedema surgery.

The process is very much like a sculptor's subtraction technique, chipping away at the fat excess diligently and purposefully until the hidden beauty reveals itself. Beautiful legs are already inside the fat mass; I just release the form. A well-aligned skeletal and a good tone of muscles determine what the ultimate result will be. Michelangelo said, "Every block of stone has a statue inside it, and it is the sculptor's task to discover it. I saw the angel in the marble and carved until I set him free."

Superdry 4D liposuction is curative liposuction that improves functionality, pain, swelling, physical appearance, and quality of life. It provides accuracy and symmetry, never achieved by other methods. This technique focuses on lymph vessel preservation as well. It eliminates the risk of fat embolization. The time when I noticed that even a perfect surgery was insufficient to handle these patients' problems led to a major improvement in my outlook toward lipoedema. The majority of lipoedema patients do not know how to eat, how to exercise, or even how to sleep well. There are so many factors that need to be addressed that may impact the postoperative outcomes. I wrote my first book on lipoedema from that point of view. It highlighted the importance of a multidisciplinary approach with plain language. However, I kept actively seeking the mystery behind lipoedema. It was the Euroke moment for me when I found its roots in the agricultural revolution and noticed that it was an evolutionary mismatch that led to writing this book.

After liposuction, I wait to pass at least three months for the second session. In most cases, I tell the patients it is a bad strategy to finish the whole lower extremity in one session. It puts you at risk. It causes more sagginess. I tell them that their metabolic rates will increase, and their appetite will reduce.

When diseased fat cells are removed through liposuction treatment, your appetite is also reduced because fewer fat cells steal all those calories. Less hunger means less overeating, which means less insulin production, which adds to long-term weight loss.

Every patient experiences a higher level of energy after the surgery. World et al. found that women with lipoedema were found to have lower resting energy expenditure. The resting energy expenditure accounts for more than 50% of the total daily energy expenditure. Total energy expenditure is the sum of resting energy expenditure, physical activity energy expenditure, and the thermic effect of food. The lower resting energy expenditure represents a slower metabolism in lipoedema.

The basal metabolic rate measures how many calories you burn while you are resting. Our body performs the most basic (basal) functions to sustain life, such as breathing, cell production, and nutrient processing. A low metabolic rate is a higher risk of gaining weight. For women – especially if you are over 40 years old – losing weight can be extra challenging. This is because of metabolic changes in your body that happen leading up to and after menopause.

As we understand the evolutionary roots of modern disease, we can develop a holistic approach to the treatment of lipoedema. Hunter-gatherer lifestyle might be a model in public health. Best management includes a multidisciplinary approach involving vascular medicine specialists, plastic surgeons, obesity and endocrinology specialists, dieticians, and physiotherapists.

A plastic surgeon should have a holistic approach. A Lipoedema Surgeon should take all of these into account: their environments, their habits, their dietary choices, and all the different treatments.

They should strive to improve every patient's quality of health. Many psychological factors impact the results of treatment besides the surgery alone. If not addressed, these psychological issues can cause a patient to be dissatisfied with the perfect surgery.

I am often asked by the patients whether or not the fat growth occurs in the other regions of their bodies.

According to the lipostatic theory proposed by Kennedy, a long-term energy balance is achieved through feedback systems that constantly regulate adipose tissue depots. Thus, an abrupt liposuction-induced decrease in body fat may trigger compensatory mechanisms that would ultimately lead to body fat regain. Although it is a risk for non-lipoedema patients to have the possible compensatory fat growth, I have never noted compensatory adipose tissue expansion at intact depots but sometimes regrowth of the fat in aspirated depots.

The novel finding of a study was that exercise training is capable of counteracting the liposuction-induced compensatory growth of visceral fat in normal-weight women (Benatti). In lipoedema patients, liposuction cannot completely remove all lipoedematous fat, and it is possible that the remaining tissue can grow over time.

Patients receiving aesthetic surgery experience a wide range of physical, psychological, and social problems. Surgery was shown to be effective at addressing these problems. Further, it has been assumed that a positive change in the patient's physical appearance will improve their psychological well-being, including their self-confidence and self-esteem.

Plastic surgery is a unique field of medicine that alleviates psychological distress through the restoration of the disfigured body. From this perspective, it would be better to call it psychoaesthetic surgery.

Teenagers with lipoedema are inherently vulnerable to comments made by others, sometimes resulting in devastating effects.

Their body changing quickly make them vulnerable. They cannot find suitable clothes like her friends, simply because of the size of her legs. The media, movies, magazines, and peers add fuel to the fire of desire for acceptance. Body shame appears to drive social isolation. This can interfere with an individual's ability to interact with classmates and teachers and may even prevent students from attending school. Forms of bullying like body shaming or fat shaming can negatively influence body image and lead to low self-esteem by deteriorating the situation much more.

In most patients, the disproportionate fat storage is already set in place in the middle of their teenage years, typically after starting their menstrual cycles. If lipoedema has already been diagnosed and there is a disproportion in place, the earlier it is targeted, the better. This will prevent it from advancing to its later stages.

One of my teenage lipoedema patients punished herself after she ate something that was said not to eat, even some fruit. The inner voice of "I shouldn't have done it." made her feel guilty. I asked her who told her not to eat fruit. She said, "A well-known doctor on TV." These kinds of things always remind me of the quote, "Those who know do not talk. Those who talk do not know." They are "blamed" for "cheating" on their prescribed diets. Most of them struggle with feelings of guilt after eating something they labeled as bad. Labeling food as good or bad prevents you from actually enjoying it. Feelings of guilt results in self-loathing, shame, and hopelessness. All contribute to eating disorders which worsen the condition. The research found that Shame and guilt are associated with eating disorder symptomatology. These emotional states may be related to binge eating because one attempts to use food to cope.

Surgeons have a pragmatic point of view. We are devoted to reaching a goal in a limited period. The handling of lipoedematous fat among our fingers, seeing the tissue layers during the lifting, touching a vein, touching a lymph channel or lymph node, and feeling how loose areolar tissue is, give us an enormous advantage in looking at lipoedema from a different point of view.

An experimental study found that the risk of lymphatic lesions is decreased by longitudinal liposuction and increased by transverse liposuction. The longitudinal technique refers to the aspiration of fat parallel to the axes of lymphatic channels. The lymphatics can tolerate longitudinal tension to some extent.

I am often asked why I don't prefer ultrasound or laser-assisted liposuction for lipoedema in the lower extremity. Lipoedematos tissue is a damaged one with an abundance of inflammatory cells. It is not convincing for me to give extra damage with thermal energy to damaged tissue. Considering the fact that even a noninvasive method, except gentle lymph drainage, might deteriorate the symptoms of lipoedema, gentle techniques should be used in lipoedema.

Excessive application of ultrasound energy can produce internal cavity formation that could lead to a seroma, even pseudobursa formation, delayed resolution of swelling, or both. Lateral movement of ultrasound-assisted liposuction cannulas or probes could produce thermal damage to deep tissues along the sides of the cannulas. In addition to prolonged tissue induration, painful dysesthesias and sensory changes caused by ultrasound injury have been reported. It has been postulated that such adverse effects result from the demyelination of sensory nerve fibers. Full-thickness skin loss and hyperpigmentation have also been reported. Ultrasound-assisted liposuction is certainly a great technique. I sometimes use it for muscle definition in the abdomen, thorax, and buttocks, but it is not for the lower legs.

# RISK EVOLUTION IN LIPOEDEMA SURGERY

I sometimes encounter catastrophic thinking in our lipoedema patients. They assume that the worst will happen in surgery. It is also known as magnifying, a kind of cognitive distortion (a thought pattern that is irrational or exaggerated). Magnifying can also affect and intensify how we experience pain. This is especially true with chronic pain patients, which can influence how patients perceive future pain. In catastrophic thinking, your brain engages your imagination and creates worst-case scenarios. It can increase anxiety and prevent people from taking action in a situation. A person in catastrophic thinking believes that various physical symptoms indicate serious health problems, even though medical tests have determined nothing is wrong.

During the consultation, some patients say, "There is no risk at all, isn't it" I always tell them. Life itself is inherently risky. Even taking antibiotics can kill you. Clostridium difficile diarrhea, anaphylactic shock, or Steven- Johnson Syndrome are some of the life-threatening complications of antibiotics.

Liposuction performed alone is a safe procedure with a low risk of major complications. The whole complication rate of liposuction is roughly 5%, with most complications being minor.

Surgical decisions aren't based upon the 'gut feeling' of the operating surgeon or anesthetist. Are you a high-risk surgical candidate or a low-risk candidate? The Surgical Risk Score assigns a numerical value to reflect the risk level associated with the procedure ranging from 1 (very low risk) to 5 (very high risk).

These categories identify operations with increased potential for substantial blood loss or other intraoperative and postoperative risks. The ASA Physical Status Classification System helps predict perioperative risks by assessing the fitness of patients. ASA 1: An average healthy patient. Example: Fit, nonobese (BMI under 30), a nonsmoking patient with good exercise tolerance.

# RESISTANCE TO BARIATRIC SURGERY

For the patients with high body mass index, I tell them they are not appropriate for safe surgery. They righteously opposed me, saying they were lipoedema patients and couldn't lose weight. They are right in terms of burning off the leg fat, but it is possible to burn off the trunk fat and reduce excess fluid in the interstitium.

I examined a woman with a body mass index of 40. She underwent a gastric sleeve operation and lost a lot of weight one year after the surgery, but her legs were slightly affected. I operated on her legs. It felt mostly fibrotic fat remained. I experienced similar tissue resistance in patients who struggled too much to lose weight with starvation diets or take diuretic plant supplements. I postulated that the interstitial space lost its fluid, but that medium made the fat hardened.

Although bariatric surgery works effectively for the obesity component, these treatments do not reduce the abnormal subcutaneous adipose tissue in the legs.

Body mass index is a simple weight-to-height ratio index commonly used in classifying overweight and obesity in adult populations and individuals. It is defined as the weight in kilograms divided by the square of the height in meters (kg m2). A body mass index greater than 25 kg m2 is considered overweight, and greater than 30 kg is considered obese. A problem with this method is that individuals with a high body mass index may be mesomorphic and have a high amount of muscle mass. Therefore, body mass index may not be the most accurate marker for total body fat percentage and an even less suitable tool to assess body fat distribution. Waist circumference is a slightly less common method used to predict obesity in an individual but may be more accurate in predicting obesity-related health issues. A waist circumference of 88 cm or greater is considered unhealthy for females.

It has become evident that total, regional, and ectopic adiposity assessments are important for predicting cardiometabolic risk, identifying the fat distribution phenotype, and for obesity treatment follow-up.

Clinical methods such as body mass index and body adiposity index make it possible to estimate total body fat but not regional adiposity; waist circumference, waist-to-hip ratio, and sagittal abdominal diameter and bioimpedance may predict or estimate abdominal fat, but do not distinguish between subcutaneous fat and visceral fat. Elevated waist circumference alone does not always identify individuals with increased visceral fat. Some authors propose that the "hypertriglyceridemic waist" that combines waist circumference and trygliceridemia values could also predict visceral obesity.

# APHRODITE REBORN

During my visit to the patients in the first postoperative period, I was usually impressed by the reactions of patients after seeing their thinned and well-shaped legs with their eyes wide open despite the fact that the effect of anesthesia did not wear off. I had an author patient who had said during the awakening of anesthesia. "Light more light, "I asked her for the meaning of these words later on. She said it was an allusion to Goethe's last words. The rumor has it that Goethe said "mehr licht" before dying. There's ongoing speculation about why he really meant it.

I had an advanced lipoedema patient from Cyprus who required two surgery sessions. I operated on the lower legs and the knee region in the first session. There months after the surgery, her surgical treatment was completed with the total upper extremity and the upper thigh liposuction. The lipocare instructions were taught, and she was sent home uneventfully. One year of the follow-up, the result was really astonishing. She totally turned to someone new. Her walking style, dressing style, posture, and energy changed.

She said she was reborn and changed her birth date to the date of her operation. This radically changed her life, and her depiction reminded me of the birth of Venus. She is also known Lady of Cyprus. The Birth of Venus, painted by Botticelli, depicts the goddess Venus arriving at the shore after her birth when she emerged from the sea fully grown. This result may sound like an extreme example, but aesthetic surgery can significantly improve the quality of life.

*"King Solomon suspected the Queen of Sheba of being Lilith because she had hairy legs. Lilith was once known as the Sumerian fertility and agricultural goddess. She protected children and helped to harvest food, but over the years has been demonified by other religions (Piiroinen).*

In the third month of follow-up, the patient was satisfied with the result and started to tell me how her complaints went away. During my examination, she apologized for the hair on her legs. She said, "Hair on her legs had disappeared after laser hair removal sessions. They came back after the lipoedema surgery.

Hair loss, reduced hair growth, and nail problems are the typical features of trophic changes in the leg due to ischemia. We can postulate that the microcirculation was restored owing to the surgery.

My hypothesis is that hair regrowth is a sign of health regeneration.

Longitudinal studies of up to eight years post-surgery have demonstrated sustained improvements in size, swelling, pain, heaviness, function, and quality of life, per my experience. Occasionally women who complain of cold feet might notice that after liposuction, there is improvement in the warmth of their toes, perhaps from more free-circulating adrenaline. Removing a lot of fat cells means there are fewer fat cells to "soak up" the insulin, adrenaline, lipases, thyroid hormone, and many other metabolites necessary to do the body's work.

# CINDERELLA'S FEET AND MY RED SOFA

I used to think that the feet are spared in lipoedema patients, and if the feet are involved, the diagnosis is lymphedema or lypolymphedema. There is some truth in it. In most patients, the upper foot below the ankle is affected. It may easily be missed when it is the subtle or thick ankle, making it invisible.

I often see lipoedema patients whose feet get bigger over time. They have difficulty putting their feet in their shoes towards the evening. During long periods of standing and/or sitting that the accumulation of fluids in the legs increases. Another less-known reason is that the additional weight may flatten the foot arch, causing an increase in shoe size. I often saw patients undergoing a liposuction procedure whose feet got smaller and narrower than before. It might be attributed to liposuction around the malleoli. Other reasons may be the spontaneous restoration of the plantar arch and less edema.

The fossil record shows that there was a big increase in leg length in early humans two million years ago. It has been suggested that one reason for this increase could have been the energy saved by having longer legs (Pontzer). Longer leg lengths have been linked with a range of adult cardiometabolic health outcomes, such as lower blood pressure and insulin resistance and reduced risk of ischemic heart disease and type 2 diabetes (Smith et al.). Liposuction helps elongate the legs, which is based on a well-known geometrical illusion. The vertical line looks longer than the same-sized horizontal line of the same length.

Most lipoedema patients ask me if they wear high heel shoes. It is an obvious question for someone who restricted the important part of their lives by avoiding wearing skirts, boots, and high heel shoes. No doubt, repressed aspirations or feelings should find a place to express themselves. I allow them on some occasions.

According to the fairy tale, Cinderella's feet perfectly fit in the glass shoes, and she and her prince lived happily ever after. I witnessed the modern adaptation of the story firsthand. In the third month of follow-up, I talked to the patient about how her lifestyle should be in accordance with lipoedema. Her shoes attracted my attention. A black ballet shoe with a rounded tip with the front strap went with the ankle-length casual black pants, exposing the tiny details of her ankle. This petite woman with a dynamic Istanbullate look started to narrate the story. She was not able to wear this size of shoes. She said it gave her enormous confidence and the feeling of freedom. Her story had allusions to the original one; not only did the feet and shoes match, but she did also live happily.

"Give a girl the correct footwear, and she can conquer the world." This quote is associated with Marilyn Monroe reminding us of a long walking scene in Niagara. Whether it is an apocryphal quote attributed to the wrong person or an anonymous one, it hides a deep philosophy inside.

It is said that Monroe aided an extra undulation of her signature walk, a more pronounced wiggle of her hips, to deepen the sway of her hip by wearing a specially altered pair of shoes, making one heel shorter than the other. No doubt, it adds to female allure on the rise of dynamic aesthetics.

The feeling of femininity is a requirement to strengthen the female identity. It is not because of Gender roles in society regarding they are expected to emphasize their femininity

The famous painting "Venus with a Mirror" shows the goddess Venus as the personification of femininity. When I highlight the importance of the aesthetic result, some women oppose me, and they say, "It is our priority to get rid of pain; we don't care about the aesthetic result." Interestingly, they change their prime concern after their symptoms disappear following the surgery and start to preoccupy with the unrealistic tiny in their legs.

This powerful feminine accessory provides a charming posture, the breasts pushing out, the buttocks sticking out, more prominent calve curvature, the increased lumbar curvature stressing the buttock curvature and elongation of the legs. The post-surgical overconfidence and elegant walking style add to these aesthetic benefits.

Based on the evolved mate preference, it can be hypothesized that high heels increase women's attractiveness via effects on their lumbar curvature.

For example, Morris et al. (2013) hypothesize that high heels increase women's attractiveness through their effects on specific biomechanical properties of women's gait.

However, wearing high heels for an extended period can increase paraspinal musculature activation of the lumbar and cervical spine, causing prolonged overload and fatigue in the trunk and neck muscles. It bears a resemblance to post-flight fatigue.

Let alone wearing the high heel shoes wrong choice of shoes can also cause a number of foot health problems, including articular, dermatological, circulatory, the Achilles tendon (which may shorten and stiffen with prolonged wear), knees (because high heels cause knees to bend constantly, which, according to some doctors, could lead to osteoarthritis later in life. Except for some occasions, events, and parties, regular and long-term high-heel shoe use is detrimental to lipoedema patients.

Impaired self-conceptualization and low self-esteem are among the main mental issues prompting patients to seek cosmetic surgery. It also holds true for lipoedema patients.

Most lipoedema patients undergo a radical shaping of their bodies not only through liposuction procedures but also through a healthy paleo lifestyle leads to it. However, they can need extra surgeries to achieve harmony in their bodies. They sometimes want me to fill their atrophic breasts from the fat aspirated from their legs. They are disappointed when I tell them there is no way to transfer the inflammatory fat to their breasts. In today's world, time is of the essence. Most people tend to squeeze a lot into their programs. They wish to have combined procedures done that are cost-effective with less downtime.

Whether it's for lipoedema or not, liposuction should always cause a little skin tightening. However, when someone has a lot of redundant loose skin, the surgeon has to be careful of how much retraction of the skin he or she is going for. After liposuction surgery, if someone already has a lot of loose skin, there may be a need for a subsequent body lifting procedure, such as a thigh lift.

In the 18th century, the French philosopher Denis Diderot wrote an essay entitled "Regrets on Parting with My Old Dressing Gown" On receiving a new dressing gown as a gift from a friend, Diderot observed that it compelled him to redecorate his entire study because the new dressing gown made everything in the room look old and shabby by comparison. He replaced his old straw chair with an armchair covered in Moroccan leather; his old desk was replaced with an expensive new writing table; his formerly beloved prints were replaced with more costly prints, and so on.

The take-home message from this anecdote is that we should get our priorities straight. No one should rush into a surgical procedure.

The discrepancy between the upper and lower body is the epitome of lipoedema.

I clearly remember a lipoedema patient with a dynamic personality and mostly self-deprecating humor. She said after the surgery, “My upper body is 40 in size, lower body 44. It was really hard to find a dress that fit me. I got rid of this annoying situation and can follow new fashion trends. Moreover, I experienced the easily sliding feeling of a skirt or dressing without resistance.”

Evidence demonstrates that cosmetic surgery improves the patient’s body image, attitude, social interactions, mental health and self-esteem, quality of life, and overall satisfaction.

Can’t say that every patient I operated on was happy. Fortunately, in just a few patients, although I shaped their legs, most of their symptoms have gone (sensitivity to pressure, complaint scores for edema, the feeling of tension score, and complaint scores for bruising were significantly reduced ), and their life quality highly increased they focused on some minor problems which are inherent of the surgical procedures such as minor asymmetries or loose tissue. They completely ignored the positive things they obtained and easily forgot their preoperative appearances. When I showed them their preoperative photos, they could not hide their surprise, saying, “Is this me?”

All-or-nothing thinking is a cognitive distortion involving the emotions such as never or ever—a negative thought process. People with this type of faulty thinking have the inability to see the real problem. For people with anxiety or depression, this often means only seeing the downside to any given situation. People who fall victim to all-or-nothing thinking believe they are either a success or a failure.

Lipoedema surgery is very demanding work. A surgeon should work in a stressful situation standing, usually for at least 4 hours. At the hospital, I operate the lipoedema patients; I sometimes meet him who is still operating. One day I asked him why he was still doing surgery. He responded by laughing, “It has always been in my mind to quit the job for ten years, but the job doesn’t give me.” In life, we should sometimes choose a career based on passion rather than money.

# THE PALEOLITHIC LIFESTYLE RELOADED

Superdry 4D liposuction for the lower legs and mid-leg and the other liposuction techniques for the remaining part are mandatory steps to break the vicious circle in lipoedema. Lipoedema certainly requires a lifestyle similar to hunter-gatherers.

It would oversimplify the situation to follow only a paleo diet. The diet you follow is not the only important thing to address in order to get healthy. It is only one aspect of the many elements. The nutritional patterns of our ancestors from the Paleolithic era differed considerably from current standards. However, there was no single Paleolithic nutritional pattern. Food choices critically depended on the geographical latitude and climate. Humans were adaptable creatures, living in contrasting environments and latitudes. Studies show that some tribes depended more on fish than plants or meat; others more on plants than meat or fish; some more on meat than fish or plants. But none consumed the prodigious quantities of sugar-based or industrialized products we enjoy today. Therefore, our Paleolithic ancestors' diets varied considerably in the composition of macronutrients and the proportion of vegetables compared with animal foods. It's clear there's no one-size-fits-all-paleo diet. Most of the fruits and vegetables we eat today have undergone profound changes through agricultural methods. You cannot easily mimic the Paleolithic diet. Selection by humans has made them larger and sweeter. Ancient man also ate plants that you can't find at a grocery store.

It is certainly true that we have inherited many adaptations from our Paleo predecessors. It is still vague which paleo diet we should follow, but there is one thing certain: the paleo lifestyle centers around how our bodies were designed to function best to act like a hunter-gatherer. No rigid, stressful diet, exercise, or anti-stress program must be followed if the behavior is adjusted based on a human being's evolutionary heritage. Returning to conditions of the Stone Age conditions is neither possible nor desirable. Paleolithic times were certainly no paradise. I remember a cartoon in which two cavemen are talking in a cave. The caption reads: 'Something's just not right – our air is clean, our water is pure, we all get plenty of exercise, everything we eat is organic and free-range, and yet nobody lives past thirty.'

Behavioral changes in eating, spontaneous physical activity, positive mental set, mindfulness, being close to nature, and re-establishing the circadian rhythm are the main elements of the paleo approach in lipoedema (Figures 14 - 15).

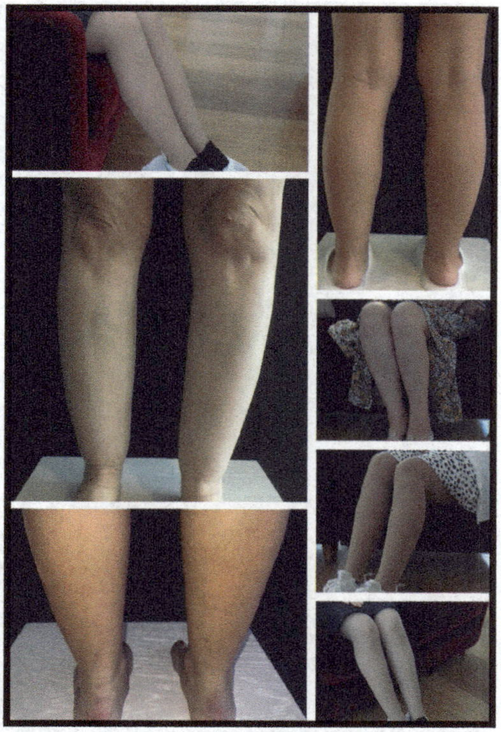

*Figure 14*

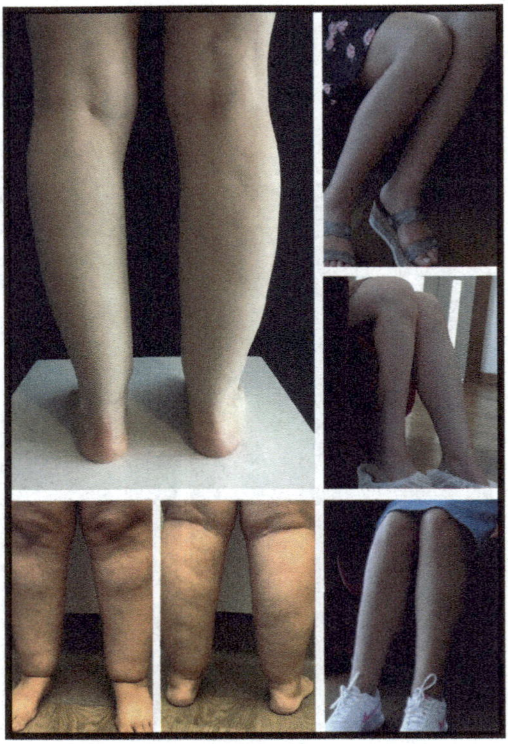

*Figure 15: Lipoedema patients in different stages. Being able to wear comfortably is among the most important proofs of the success of the procedure.*

# REFERENCES


Abraham, S., Tschanz, C., Krischer, J., Saurat, J.H. (2007). "Lymphangitis due to insect sting" Dermatology 215: 260–261.

Abramson, J.H., Hopp, C., Epstein, L.M. (1981). "The epidemiology of varicose veins. A survey in western Jerusalem" J Epidemiol Comm Health 35:213-217Beaglehole, R. (1986). "Epidemiology of Varicose Veins" World J. Surg. 10: 898-902.

Abtahian, F. vd. (2003). "Regulation of blood and lymphatic vascular separation by signaling proteins SLP-76 and Syk" Science 299: 247–251

Adair, T.H., Moffatt, D.S., Paulsen, A.W., Guyton, A.C. (1982). "Quantitation of changes in lymph protein concentration during lymph node transit" Am J Physiol 243: H351-H359

Adair, T.H., Guyton, A.C. (1983). "Modification of lymph by lymph nodes. II. Effect of increased lymph node venous blood pressure" Am J Physiol 245: H616-H622

Adair, T.H., Guyton, A.C. (1985). "Modification of lymph by lymph nodes. III. Effect of increased lymph hydrostatic pressure" Am J Physiol 249: H777-H782

Adler, C.J. vd. (2013). "Sequencing ancient calcified dental plaque shows changes in oral microbiota with dietary shifts of the Neolithic and Industrial revolutions" Nature Genetics, 45(4), 450–455.

Agullo, F.J., Palladino, H., Sozer, S.O., Nikolay, S. (2017). "Complications of liposuction, advanced techniques in liposuction and fat transfer" Available at http://www.intechopen.com/books/advanced-techniques-in-liposuction-and Accessed at 15 May 2017

Ahima, R., Flier, J. (2000). "Adipose tissue as an endocrine organ" *Trends Endocrinol Metab* 11: 327–332.

Ajamian, M., Steer, D., Rosella, G. vd. (2019). "Serum zonulin as a marker of intestinal mucosal barrier function: May not be what it seems" *PLoS One.* 14(1): e0210728. https://doi.org/10.1371/journal.pone.0210728

Al-Ghadban, S. vd. (2019). "Dilatedblood and lymphatic microvessels, angiogenesis, increased macrophages, and adipocyte hypertrophy in lipedema thigh skin and fat tissue" Journal of Obesity. 8747461

Al-Ghadban, S., Herbst, L., Bunnell, B.A. (2019). "Lipedema: A Painful Adipose Tissue Disorder, Adipose Tissue - An Update" Leszek Szablewski, IntechOpen, Doi: 10.5772/intechopen.88632. Available from: https://www.intechopen.com/books/adipose-tissue-an-update/lipedema-a-painful-adipose-tissue-disorder

Alboni, P., Alboni, M., Bertorelle, G. (2008). "The origin of vasovagal syncope: to protect the heart or to escape predation?" Clin Auton Res. Aug; 18(4): 170-8.

Allen, E.V., Hines, E.A. (1940). "Lipedema of the legs: a syndrome characterized by fat legs and orthostatic edema" Proc Staff Meet Mayo Clin. 15:184–187

Altay, F., Karbancıoğlu-Güler, F., Daskaya-Dikmen, C., Heperkan, D. (2013). "A review on traditional Turkish fermented non-alcoholic beverages: microbiota, fermentation process and quality characteristics" Int J Food Microbiol. Oct 1;167(1): 44-56.

Alwardat, N. vd. (2019) "The effect of lipedema on health-related quality of life and psychological status: a narrative review of the literature" *Eating and Weight Disorders*: 1-6.

Amann-Vesti, B.R., Franzeck, U.K., Bollinger, A. (2001). "Microlymphatic aneurysms in patients with lipedema" *Lymphology.* 34: 170–175.

Amiot, M.J. vd. (2016). "Effects of dietary polyphenols on metabolic syndrome features in humans: a systematic review" Obes. Rev. 17: 573-586

Amsler, F., Blattler, W. (2008). "Compression therapy for occupational leg symptoms and chronic venous disorders—A meta-analysis of randomised controlled trials" Eur J Vasc Endovasc Surg 35:366–372

Anderson, J.W., Konz, E.C., Frederich, R.C., Wood, C.L. (2001). "Long-term weight-loss maintenance: a meta-analysis of U.S. studies" *Am J Clin Nutr* 74: 579–584

Anderson, N.D., Lau, M.A., Segal, Z.V., Bishop, S.R. (2007). "Mindfulness-based stress reduction and attentional control" *Clin. Psychol. Psychother.* 14:449. doi: 10.1002/cpp.544

Anderson, V. (2004). "Creatures of Empire: How Domestic Animals Transformed Early America" New York: Oxford University Press, 32-35

Anh, N.H., Kim, S.J., Long, N.P. vd. (2020). "Ginger on Human Health: A Comprehensive Systematic Review of 109 Randomized Controlled Trials" Nutrients 12(1):157.

Armelagos, G.J. vd. (1989). "The origins of agriculture" Mark Nathan Cohen, Health and the rise of civilization (New Haven: Con.), 61-2, 115-117

Armelagos, G.J. (1991). "Population Growth during a Period of Declining Health" Population and Environment, 13(1): 9-22.

Arnoldi, C.C. (1964). "The venous return from the lower leg: a synthesis" *Acta Orthop Scand.* 64: 1–75

Aukland, K. (1994). "Why don't our feet swelling in the upright position?" News Physiol Sci 9: 214–219.

Aydın, M.A., Salukhe, T.V., Wilke, I., Willems, S. (2010). "Management and therapy of vasovagal syncope: A review" World J Cardiol. Oct 26; 2(10): 308-15

Babic, T., Browning, K.N. (2014). "The role of vagal neurocircuits in the regulation of nausea and vomiting" Eur J Pharmacol 722: 38–47

Baddour, L.M., Bisno, A.L. (1985). "Non-group A beta-hemolytic streptococcal cellulitis: association with venous and lymphatic compromise" Am J Med. 79:155–159.

Badman, M.K., Flier, J.S. (2005). "The gut and energy balance: visceral allies in the obesity wars" Science 307:1909–1914

Baranowska, B., Bik, W. (2010). "Fizjologiczna rola adiponektyny" *Postep Nauk Med* 6: 503–508

Bates, V. (2016). "'Under Cross-Examination She Fainted': Sexual Crime and Swooning in the Victorian Courtroom" *Journal of Victorian Culture,* 21:4, 456-470,

Bauer, A.T. vd. (2019). "New Insights on Lipedema" *Plastic and Reconstructive Surgery.* 144(6): 1475

Baumgartner, A., Hueppe, M., Schmeller, W. (2016). "Long-term benefit of liposuction in patients with lipoedema: a follow-up study after an average of 4 and 8 years" Br J Dermatol. 174(5):1061–1067.

Baxter, R.A. (1999). "Histologic effects of ultrasound-assisted lipoplasty" *Aesthetic Surg* J 19:109–114.

Baviera, G. vd. (2014). "Microbiota in healthy skin and in atopic eczema" Biomed Res Int 436921.

Bazar, K.A., Yun, A.J., Lee, P.Y. (2004). "Debunking a myth: neurohormonal and vagal modulation of sleep centers, not redistribution of blood flow, may account for postprandial somnolence" *Med Hypotheses*. 63(5):778-782

Beaglehole, R., Prior, I.A.M., Salmond, C.E., Davidson, F. (1975). "Varicose veins in the South Pacific" Int J. Epidemiol. 4: 295-99.

Bechara, F.G., vd. (2006). "Lipolysis of lipomas in patients with familial multiple lipomatosis: an ultrasonography-controlled trial" *J Cutan Med Surg.* 10:155–159

Becker, C., Neurath, M.F., Wirtz, S. (2015). "The intestinal microbiota in inflammatory bowel disease" ILAR J 56:192–204

Beighton, P.H. vd. (1988). "International nosology of heritable disorders of connective tissue, Berlin 1986" *Am J Med Genet* 29: 581–594

Beja-Pereira, A. vd. (2006). "The origin of European cattle: evidence from modern and ancient DNA" *Proc Natl Acad Sci U S A* 103: 8113-8118.

Belcaro, G., Nicolaides, A.N. (2000). *Noninvasive Investigations in Vascular Disease*, Imperial College Press, London

Beltran, K., Herbst, K. L. (2017). "Differentiating lipedema and dercum's disease" International Journal of Obesity, vol. 41, no. 2, pp. 240–245

Benatti, F. vd. (2012). "Liposuction Induces a Compensatory Increase of Visceral Fat Which Is Effectively Counteracted by Physical Activity: A Randomized Trial" The Journal of Clinical Endocrinology & Metabolism, Volume 97, Issue 7, 1 July 2012, Pages 2388–2395

Benedik, E. (2022). "Sources of vitamin D for humans" Int J Vitam Nutr Res. Mar; 92(2): 118-125

Benigni, J.P., Sadoun, S., Allaert, F.A. vd. (2003). "Efficacy of class 1 elastic compression stockings in the early stages of chronic venous disease. A comparative study" *Int Angiol* 22: 383–392

Bennion, L.D., Adams, G.R. (1986). "A revision of the extended version of the objective measure of ego identity status: An identity instrument for use with late adolescents" Journal of Adolescent Research, 1, 183-198.

Bermon S. vd. (2015). "The microbiota: an exercise immunology perspective" Exercise Immunology Review. 21: 70–79.

Berthoud, H-R. (2008). "The vagus nerve, food intake and obesity" Regul Pept 149: 15–25

Bilancini, S., Lucchi, M., Tucci, S., Eleuteri, P. (1995). "Functional lymphatic alterations in patients suffering from lipedema" *Angiology* 46: 333-339.

Bilgiç, H., Hakkı, E.E., Pandey, A., Khan, M.K., Akkaya, M.S. (2016). "Ancient DNA from 8400 Year-Old Çatalhöyük Wheat: Implications for the Origin of Neolithic Agriculture" PLoS One. Mar 21; 11(3): e0151974.

Bird-David, N. (1992). "Beyond 'the original affluent society': a culturalist reformulation" Current Anthropol. 33(1): 25–47. doi: 10.1086/204029.

Bishehsari, F., Voigt, R.M., Keshavarzian, A. (2020). "Circadian rhythms and the gut microbiota: from the metabolic syndrome to cancer" *Nat Rev Endocrinol* 16, 731–739

Björntorp, P. (1991). "Metabolic implications of body fat distribution" *Diabetes Care* 14: 1132–1143

Bilancini, S. vd. (1995). "Functional lymphatic alterations in patients suffering from lipedema" *Angiology* 46: 333-339

Bogaard, A. vd. (2013). "Crop manuring and intensive land management by Europe's first farmers" *Proc Natl Acad Sci U S A* 110: 12589-12594

Bogaard, A. vd. (2013). "The archaeobotany of mid-later occupation levels at Çatalhöyük" *Humans and Landscapes of Çatalhöyük: Reports from the 2000-2008 Seasons*, editor Ian Hodder, Cotsen Institute of Archaeology Press, Los Angeles, CA vol. 8, 93–128

Bogaard, A. vd. (2017). "Agricultural innovation and resilience in a long-lived early farming community: The 1,500-year sequence at Neolithic Çatalhöyük, central Anatolia" *Anatol. Stud.* 67, 1–28

Bollinger, A., Amann-Vesti, B.R. (2007). "Fluorescence microlymphography: diagnostic potential in lymphedema and basis for the measurement of lymphatic pressure and flow velocity" *Lymphology*. 40: 52–62.

Bolton, M.A., Pruzinsky, T., Cash, T.F., & Persing, J.A. (2003). "Measuring outcomes in plastic surgery: Body image and quality of life in abdominoplasty patients" Plastic & Reconstructive Surgery, 112, 619-625.

Bonaz, B., Sinniger, V., Pellissier, S. (2016). "Anti-inflammatory properties of the vagus nerve: potential therapeutic implications of vagus nerve stimulation" J Physiol 594:5781–5790

Bonaz, B., Bazin, T., Pellissier, S. (2018). "The Vagus Nerve at the Interface of the Microbiota-Gut-Brain Axis" Front Neurosci. Feb 7;12:49. doi: 10.3389/fnins.2018.00049. PMID: 29467611; PMCID: PMC5808284.

Bosman, E.S., Albert, A.Y., Lui, H., Dutz, J.P., Vallance, B.A. (2019). "Skin exposure to narrow band ultraviolet (UVB) light modulates the human intestinal microbiome" Front Microbiol. 10: 2410.

Bouchard, C. vd. (1990). "The response to long-term overfeeding in identical twins" *N Engl J Med* 322: 1477–1482

Bouchard, C., Despres, J.P., Mauriege, P. (1993) "Genetic and nongenetic determinants of regional fat distribution" *Endocr Rev* 14: 72–93

Boulenger, J.P., Uhde, T.W., Wolff, E.A., III, Post, R.M. (1984). "Increased sensitivity to caffeine in patients with panic disorders" *Arch Gen Psychiatry* 41: 1067–1071

Brand, F.N., Dannenberg, A.L., Abbott, R.D., Kannel, W.B. (1988). "The epidemiology of varicose veins: The Framingham study" Am J Prev Med 4: 96-101.

Bray, M.S., Young, M.E. (2007). "Circadian rhythms in the development of obesity: potential role for the circadian clock within the adipocyte" *Obes Rev.* Mar;8(2):169-181

Bräutigam, P. vd. (1998). "Analysis of lymphatic drainage in various forms of leg edema using two compartment lymphoscintigraphy" *Lymphology* 31: 43-55

Breneman, J.C. (1978). "Basics of food allergy" *Springfield, IL*: Charles C. Thomas; 8

Brenner, S.L. vd. (2015). "Evolutionary Mismatch and Chronic Psychological Stress" *Journal of Evolutionary Medicine,* Ashdin Publishing, vol.3, doi: 10.4303/jem/235885

Breu, F.X., Wollmann, J.C. (2010). "Clinical and technical follow-up after sclerotherapy" *Dermatol Surg.* 36(Suppl 2): 1004–1009. doi: 10.1111/j.1524-4725.2009.01404.x.

Bringhurst, F.R., Demay, M.B. and Kronenberg, H.M. (2003). "Hormones and Disorders of Mineral Metabolism" In: Larsen, P.R., Kronenberg, H.M., Melmed, S., et al., Eds., Williams Textbook of Endocrinology, 10th Edition, Elsevier, Philadelphia, 1323-1324.

Britto, S., Kellermayer, R. (2019). "Carbohydrate Monotony as Protection and Treatment for Inflammatory Bowel Disease" *J Crohns Colitis.* 25;13(7): 942-948.

Brockington, G. vd. (2021). "Storytelling increases oxytocin and positive emotions and decreases cortisol and pain in hospitalized children" Proc Natl Acad Sci U S A. Jun 1; 118(22): e2018409118

Brorson, H., Ohlin, K., Olsson, G., Svensson, B., Svensson, H. (2008). "Controlled compression and liposuction treatment for lower extremity lymphedema" *Lymphology.* 41:52–63

Brown, E.A. (2012). "Genetic explorations of recent human metabolic adaptations: hypotheses and evidence" Biological Reviews. 87: 838–855.

Brown, R.G. (2016). "The book of Lilith" Google books, p. 210

Browning, K.N., Verheijden, S., Boeckxstaens, G.E. (2017). "The vagus nerve in appetite regulation, mood, and intestinal inflammation" Gastroenterology 152:730–744

Bruce, M., Scott, N., Shine, P., Lader, M. (1992). "Anxiogenic effects of caffeine in patients with anxiety disorders" *Arch Gen Psychiatry* 49: 867–869

Buck, D.W., Herbst, K.L. (2016). "Lipedema: a relatively common disease with extremely common misconceptions" *Plast Reconstr Surg Glob Open.* 4(9): e1043

Burkitt, D.P. (1972). "Varicose veins, deep vein thrombosis, and haemorrhoids: Epidemiology and suggested aetiology" BMJ 2: 556-561.

Burkitt, D.P. (1976). "Varicose veins: facts and fantasies" Arch Surg 111: 1327-1332.

Buso, G. vd. (2019). "Lipedema: A Call to Action!" *Obesity (Silver Spring)* Oct; 27(10): 1567–1576

Callam, M.J., Ruckley, C.V., Dale, J.J. vd. (1987). "Hazards of compression treatment of the leg: an estimate from Scottish surgeons" *Br Med J (Clin Res Ed)* 295: 1382

Campbell, A., *Matthews*, S. (2005). "Darwin'*s illness revealed*" Postgrad Med J. Apr; 81(954): 248–251. doi: 10.1136/pgmj.2004.025569

Campbell, P.J., Carlson, M.G., Hill, J.O., Nurjhan, N. (1992). "Regulation of free fatty acid metabolism by insulin in humans: role of lipolysis and reesterification" *Am. J. Physiol.* 263(6 Pt 1), 1063–1069

Cannon, W.B. (1927). *Bodily Changes in Pain, Hunger, Fear and Rage: An Account of Recent Researches into the Function of Emotional Excitement,* D. Appleton and Company, New York, USA.

Canoy, D. vd. (2005). "Cigarette smoking and fat distribution in 21, 828 British men and women: a population-based study" Obes Res 13:1466–1475.

Capron, J.P., Delamarre, J., Herve, M.A. vd. (1981). "Meal frequency and duration of overnight fast: a role in gall-stone formation?" *Br Med J.* 283: 1435

Carabotti, M., Scirocco, A., Maselli, M.A., Severi, C. (2015). "The gut-brain axis: interactions between enteric microbiota, central and enteric nervous systems" Ann Gastroenterol 28: 203–209.

Cárdenas-Camarena, L., Arenas-Quintana, R., Robles-Cervantes, J.A. (2011). "Buttocks fat grafting: 14 years of evolution and experience" Plast Reconstr Surg. 128:545–555

Cárdenas-Camarena, L., Bayter, J.E., Aguirre-Serrano, H. vd. (2015). "Deaths caused by gluteal lipoinjection: what are we doing wrong?" Plast Reconstr Surg. 136:58–66

Carlberg, C. (2019). "Nutrigenomics of Vitamin D" Nutrients. Mar 21;11(3): 676.

Carter, C.S. (2018). "Oxytocin and Human Evolution" Curr Top Behav Neurosci. 35: 291-319.

Carvalho, C.A. vd. (2015). "Reduction of Pain and Edema of the Legs by Walking Wearing Elastic Stockings" Int J Vasc Med. 648074. doi: 10.1155/2015/648074

Chang, Q., Liu, R., Shen, Z. (2013). "Effects of slow breathing rate on blood pressure and heart rate variabilities" Int. J. Cardiol. 169: e6–e8.

Charles, M. vd. (2014). "Landscape and taskscape at Çatalhöyük: An integrative perspective" *Integrating Çatalhöyük: Themes from the 2000-2008 Seasons*, editor Ian Hodder, Cotsen Institute of Archaeology Press, Los Angeles, CA, 71–108

Charon, R. (2006). "Narrative medicine" *Honoring the stories of illness* Oxford University Press, New York.

Charon, R. (2001). "Narrative medicine: A model for empathy, reflection, profession, and trust" *JAMA* Oct 17; 286(15): 1897–902

Charon, R., Hermann, N., Devlin, M.J. (2016). "Close reading and creative writing in clinical education: teaching attention, representation, and affiliation" *Acad Med.* 91(3): 345–350

Chen, K., Xie, Y., Hu, P., Zhao, S., Mo, Z. (2010). "Multiple symmetric lipomatosis: substantial subcutaneous adipose tissue accumulation did not induce glucose and lipid metabolism dysfunction" *Ann Nutr Metab.* 57(1): 68–73

Chenard, C.A., Rubenstein, L.M., Snetselaar, L.G., Wahls, T.L. (2019). "Nutrient

Composition Comparison between a Modified Paleolithic Diet for Multiple Sclerosis and the Recommended Healthy U.S.-Style Eating Pattern" Nutrients. Mar 01; 11(3)

Child, A.H., Gordon, K.D., Sharpe, P. vd. (2010). "Lipedema: an inherited condition" Am J Med Genet A 152A: 970-976.

Chiu, K.L. vd. (2006). "Effects of venous compression of the legs on overnight rostral fluid shift and obstructive sleep apnea" Am J Respir Crit Care Med. Dec 15; 174(12): 1378-83.

Chow, J. (2002). "Probiotics and prebiotics: A brief overview" J Ren Nutr. Apr;12(2): 76-86. doi: 10.1053/jren.2002.31759. PMID: 11953920.

Christen, A.G., Christen, J.A. (1997). "Horace Fletcher (1849-1919): 'The Great Masticator'" *J Hist Dent.* Nov; 45(3): 95-100

Clavel T. vd. (2005). "Intestinal bacterial communities that produce active estrogen-like compounds enterodiol and enterolactone in humans" Appl. Environ. Microbiol. 71: 6077-6085

Clayes, R., Thiery, L., Uytterhaegen, P. (1993). "La pompe musculaire du mollet: videophlebographie et EMG simultanée" *Phlébologie* 46: 287–292

Colberg, S.R. vd. (2009). "Postprandial walking is better for lowering the glycemic effect of dinner than pre-dinner exercise in type 2 diabetic individuals" *J Am Med Dir Assoc.* 10(6):394 - 397

Collins, P.S. vd. (1989). "Abnormalities of lymphatic drainage in lower extremities: a lymphoscintigraphic study" J Vasc Surg. 9: 145–152.

Comiskey, C. (2004). "Cosmetic Surgery in Paris in 1926: The Case of the Amputated Leg" Journal of Women's History. Vol. 16, Iss. 3; 26-30

Cordain, L. (1999). "Cereal grains: Humanity's double-edged sword" World Review of Nutrition and Dietetics, 84, 19–73.

Coetzee, O., Filatova, D. (2017). "Lipidema and Lymphedema: the 'Leaky Lymph,' Weight Loss Resistance and the Intestinal Permeability Connection" EC Nutrition 11.6, 233-243.

Cogen, A.L., Nizet, V., Gallo, R.L. (2008). "Skin microbiota: a source of disease or defence?" Br J Dermatol. 158(3): 442-455

Coon, W.W., Willis, P.W., Keller, J.B. (1973). "Venous thromboembolism and other venous disease in the Tecumseh Community Health Study" Circulation 48: 839-846.

Cornu-Thenard, A., Boivin, P., Baud, J-M., de Vincenzi, I., Carpentier, P.H. (1994). "Importance of the familial factor in varicose disease: Clinical study of 134 families" J Dermatol Surg Oncol 20: 318-326.

Cox, N.H. (2002). "Management of lower leg cellulitis" Clin Med (Lond) 2:23–27

Craven, M.P., Fekete, E.M. (2019). "Weight-related shame and guilt, intuitive eating, and binge eating in female college students" Eat Behav. 33: 44-48.

Crawford, M.A., Gale, M.M., Woodford, M.H. (1969). "Linoleic acid and linolenic acid elongation products in muscle tissue of Syncerus caffer and other ruminant species" Biochem J 115: 25-27.

Crerand, C.E., Franklin, M., Sarwer, D.B. (2008). "Body dysmorphic disorder and cosmetic surgery" Plastic & Reconstructive Surgery, 122, 1-15.

Curri, S.B., Merlen, J.F. (1986). "Microvascular disorders of adipose tissue" *J Mal Vasc.* 11: 303-309

Curry, F.E., Huxley, V.H., Adamson, R.H. (1983). "Permeability of single capillaries to intermediate-sized colored solutes" Am J Physiol, 245: H495-H505

Çelik, E.E., Gökmen, V. (2018). "A Study on Interactions between the Insoluble Fractions of Different Coffee Infusions and Major Cocoa Free Antioxidants and Different Coffee Infusions and Dark Chocolate" Food Chem. 255, 8–14.

Dadras, S.S. vd. (2005). "Tumor lymphangiogenesis predicts melanoma metastasis to sentinel lymph nodes" Mod Pathol 18: 1232–1242

Dadras, M., Mallinger, P.J., Corterier, C.C., Theodosiadi, S., Ghods, M. (2017). "Liposuction in the treatment of lipedema: a longitudinal study" Arch Plast Surg. 44(4): 324–331.

Dafni, H., Israely, T., Bhujwalla, Z.M., Benjamin, L.E., Neeman, M. (2002). "Overexpression of vascular endothelial growth factor 165 drives peritumor interstitial convection and induces lymphatic drain: magnetic resonance imaging, confocal microscopy, and histological tracking of triple-labeled albumin" Cancer Res 62: 6731–6739

Dalal, A., (2017). "Interventions for the prevention of recurrent erysipelas and cellulitis"

Cochrane Database Syst Rev (6): CD009758

D'Angelo, A., Selhub, J. (1997). "Homocystine and thrombotic disease" Blood 90: 1-11.

Date, Y. (2014). "The vagus nerve and ghrelin function. Central Functions of the Ghrelin Receptor: The Receptors" New York, NY: Springer; p. 53–61.

Date, Y. (2012). "Ghrelin and the vagus nerve" Methods Enzymol 514:261–269

Davis, G. Senger, D.R. (2005). "Endothelial Extracellular Matrix: Biosynthesis, Remodeling, and Functions During Vascular Morphogenesis and Neovessel Stabilization" Circ Res 97: 1093–1107

Davis, G.E. (2009). "Matricryptic sites control tissue injury responses in the cardiovascular system: Relationships to pattern recognition receptor regulated events" J Mol Cel Cardiol in press, 454-460

De Benedetto, M.A.C., de Castro, A.G., de Carvalho, E., Sanogo, R., Blasco, P.G. (2007). "From suffering to transcendence. Narratives in palliative care" *Can Fam Physician.* 53: 1277–1279

De Filippo, C. vd. (2010). "Impact of diet in shaping gut microbiota revealed by a comparative study in children from europe and rural Africa" *Proc. Natl. Acad. Sci. U.S.A.* 107 14691–14696 10.1073/pnas.1005963107

Deby, C. (1989). "Decreased tocopherol concentrations of varicose veins associated with a decrease in antilipoperoxidant activity without similar changes in plasma" Phlebology 4: 113.

Del Rosso, James, Q. Levin, Jacqueline (2011). "The Clinical Relevance of Maintaining the Functional Integrity of the Stratum Corneum in both Healthy and Disease-affected Skin". The Journal of Clinical and Aesthetic Dermatology. 4 (9): 22–42.

DePhillipo, N.N. vd. (2018). "Efficacy of Vitamin C Supplementation on Collagen Synthesis and Oxidative Stress After Musculoskeletal Injuries: A Systematic Review" Orthop J Sports Med. Oct 25; 6(10): 2325967118804544.

Descartes, R. (1991). Principles of Philosophy, Kluwer Academic Publisher.

Després, J.P. (2012). "Body fat distribution and risk of cardiovascular disease: an update" *Circulation* 126(10): 1301–1313

Diamond, J. (1997). *Guns, Germs, and Steel: The Fates of Human Societies*, W.W. Norton, New York.

Diehl, R.R. (2005). "Vasovagal syncope and Darwinian fitness" Clin Auton Res. Apr; 15(2): 126-129.

Dietrich, O., Notroff, J. (2015). "A sanctuary, or so fair a house? In defense of an archaeology of cult at Pre-Pottery Neolithic Göbekli Tepe" In: Nicola Laneri (eds.), Defining the Sacred: Approaches to the Archaeology of Religion in the Near East. Oxford: Oxbow 75-89.

Dietrich, O., Notroff, J., Schmidt, K. (2017). "Feasting, Social Complexity and the Emergence of the Early Neolithic of Upper Mesopotamia: A View from Göbekli Tepe" in:

R. J. Chacon and R. G. Mendoza (eds.), Feast, Famine or Fighting? Multiple Pathways to Social Complexity. Studies in Human Ecology and Adaptation 8, New York: Springer 91-132.

Dietzel, R., Reisshauer, A., Jahr, S., Calafiore, D., Armbrecht, G. (2015). "Body composition in lipoedema of the legs using dual-energy X-ray absorptiometry: a case-control study" *Br J Dermatol* 173: 594-596.

Dimidi, E., Cox, S.R., Rossi, M., Whelan, K. (2019). "Fermented Foods: Definitions and Characteristics, Impact on the Gut Microbiota and Effects on Gastrointestinal Health and Disease" Nutrients. Aug 5; 11(8): 1806. doi: 10.3390/nu11081806. PMID: 31387262; PMCID: PMC6723656

Dinges, W.L. vd. (2005). "Regional body fat distribution in HIV-infected patients with lipodystrophy" *J Investig Med.* 53(1): 15–25

DiNicolantonio, J.J., O'Keefe, J.H., Wilson, W. (2018). "Subclinical magnesium deficiency: a principal driver of cardiovascular disease and a public health crisis" Open Heart. Jan 13; 5(1): e000668.

Distante, F., Bacci, P.A., Carrera, M. (2006). "Efficacy of a multifunctional plant complex in the treatment of the so-called 'cellulite': clinical and instrumental evaluation" *Int J Cosmet Sci.* 28(3): 191-206.

Dixon, J.B. (2010). "Lymphatic lipid transport: sewer or subway?" Trends Endocrinol Metab.

Divinsky, M. (2007). "Stories for life. Introduction to narrative medicine" *Can Fam Physician.* 53: Eng. 203–204, Fr. 209–211

Do, M.T., Chang, V.C., Kuran, N., Thompson, W. (2015). "Fall-related injuries among Canadian seniors, 2005–2013: an analysis of the Canadian Community Health Survey" Chronic Dis. Inj. Can. 35, 99

Doyal, L. (1991). *The Political Economy of Health*, Pluto Press

Du Preez, S., Corbitt, M., Cabanas, H. vd. (2018). "A systematic review of enteric dysbiosis in chronic fatigue syndrome/myalgic encephalomyelitis" *Systematic Reviews,* volume 7, Article number: 241

Du Teil, E.M. vd. (2018). "Talk to your gut: the oral-gut microbiome axis and its immunomodulatory role in the etiology of rheumatoid arthritis" FEMS Microbiol. Rev.

Dubnov-Raz, G., Constantini, N.W., Yariv, H., Nice, S., Shapira, N. (2011). "Influence of water drinking on resting energy expenditure in overweight children" *Int J Obes (Lond).* 35(10): 1295-1300.

Dupuy, A. vd. (1999). "Risk factors for erysipelas of the leg (cellulitis): case-control study" BMJ. 318:1591–1594.

Duarte, I.C. vd. (2017). "Tribal love: the neural correlates of passionate engagement in football fans" Soc Cogn Affect Neurosci. May 1; 12(5): 718-728

Ducimetiere, P., Richard, J.L., Pequignot, G., Warnett, J.M. (1981). "Varicose veins: A risk factor for atherosclerotic disease in middle-aged men" Int J Epidem 10: 329-335.

Dunbar, R. (2014). "How conversations around campfires came to be" Proceedings of the National Academy of Sciences 111 (39) 14013-14014. Sept.22 DOI:10.1073/pnas.1416382111

Dye, S.F. (1987). "An evolutionary perspective of the knee" J Bone Joint Surg Am. Sep; 69(7): 976-83.

Eaton, S.B., Konner, M.J. (1985). "Paleolithic nutrition. A consideration of its nature and current implications" N Engl J Med 312: 283-289.

Ebbeling, C.B. vd. (2012). "Effects of dietary composition on energy expenditure during weight-loss maintenance" *JAMA* 307: 2627-2634

Ebbeling, C.B., Feldman, H.A., Klein, G.L. vd. (2018). "Effects of a low carbohydrate diet on energy expenditure during weight loss maintenance: randomized trial" *BMJ* 363: k4583, Nov 14, doi: 10.1136/bmj.k4583

Eikelboom, J.W, Baker, R.I. (1998). "Venous thrombosis and hyperhomocysteinaemia" MJA 169: 313-315.

Eklof, B. vd. (2004). "Revision of the CEAP classification for chronic venous disorders: consensus statement" *Journal of Vascular Surgery* 40(6):1248-1252.

El-Bendary, N., Tan, Q., Pivot, F.C., Lam, A. (2013). "Fall detection and prevention for the elderly: A review of trends and challenges" Int. J. Smart Sens. Intell. Syst. 6, 1230–1266

Elfhag, K., Rössner, S. (2005). "Who succeeds in maintaining weight loss? A conceptual review of factors associated with weight loss maintenance and weight regain" *Obes. Rev.* 6:67–85. doi: 10.1111/j.1467-789X.2005.00170.x

Emanuele, E., Bertona, M., Geroldi, D. (2010). "A multilocus candidate approach identifies ACE and HIF1A as susceptibility genes for cellulite" *J Eur Acad Dermatol Venereol* 24: 930–935

Emanuele, E., Minoretti, P., Altabas, K. vd. (2011). "Adiponectin expression in subcutaneous adipose tissue is reduced in women with cellulite" *Int J Dermatol* 50: 412–416

Eneroth, H., Wallin, S., Leander, K., Nilsson Sommar, J., Åkesson, A. (2017). "Risks and Benefits of Increased Nut Consumption: Cardiovascular Health Benefits Outweigh the Burden of Carcinogenic Effects Attributed to Aflatoxin B- Exposure" Nutrients. Dec 13; 9(12): 1355. doi: 10.3390/nu9121355. PMID: 29236075; PMCID: PMC5748805.

Epstein, L.H., Temple, J.L., Roemmich, J.N., Bouton, M.E. (2009). "Habituation as a determinant of human food intake" *Psychol Rev* 116:384–407

Eriksson, H. vd. (1995). "Evidence for the key role of the adipocyte cGMP-inhibited cAMP phosphodiesterase in the antilipolytic action of insulin" *Biochim. Biophys. Acta* 1266(1), 101–107

Eshed, V., Gopher, A., Pinhasi, R., Hershkovitz, I. (2010). "Paleopathology and the Origin of Agriculture in the Levant" American Journal o fPhysical Anthropology, 143: 121-133.

Ewald, P. (1994). *Evolution of Infectious Disease,* Oxford University Press, New York

Ewald, P.W. (1980). "Evolutionary biology and the treatment of signs and symptoms of infectious disease" *J Theor Biol* 86: 169-176

Ewald, P.W. (1995). "The evolution of virulence: a unifying link between ecology and parasitology" *J Parasitol* 81: 659-669

Ewart, A., Perry, C., Connell, J. vd. (2004). "The role of insulin and the adipocytokines in regulation of vascular endothelial function" *Clin Sci* 107: 519–532

Evans, R.D.R., Antonelou, M., Henderson, S., Walsh, S.B., Salama, A.D. (2019). "Emerging evidence of an effect of salt on innate and adaptive immunity" *Nephrol. Dial. Transplant.* Dec 01;34(12):2007-2014.

Fabbrini, E., Sullivan, S., Klein, S. (2010). "Obesity and nonalcoholic fatty liver disease: biochemical, metabolic, and clinical implications" *Hepatology* 51(2): 679–689.

Faerber, G. (2014). "Der übergewichtige Patient mit CVI oder Lymphödem. Risikofaktor oder Ursache?" *Vasomed* 26: 19

Faraj, M., Lu, H., Cianflone, K. (2004). "Diabetes, lipids, and adipocyte secretagogues" *Biochem Cell Biol.* 82: 170–190

Farshchi, H.R., Taylor, M.A., Macdonald, I.A. (2004). "Regular meal frequency creates more appropriate insulin sensitivity and lipid profiles compared with irregular meal frequency in healthy lean women" *Eur J Clin Nutr.* 58: 1071–1077

Febbraio, M.A., Pedersen, B.K. (2005). "Contraction-induced myokine production and release: is skeletal muscle an endocrine organ?" *Exercise and Sport Sciences Reviews* 33: 114-119.

Ferraro, G.A., Rossano, F., Andrea, F. (2005). "Self-perception and self-esteem of patients Seeking Cosmetic Surgery" Aesthetic Plastic Surgery, 103, 83-89.

Ferreira, J.J. vd. (2010). "Manual lymphatic drainage for premenstrual syndrome symptoms: a pilot study" Fisioter Pesq. 17: 75–80.

Fielding, J.M., Rowley, K.G., Cooper, P., O' Dea, K. (2005). "Increases in plasma lycopene concentration after consumption of tomatoes cooked with olive oil" Asia Pac J Clin Nutr. 14(2):131-136.

Fife, C.E., Maus, E.A., Carter, M.J. (2010). "Lipedema: a frequently misdiagnosed and misunderstood fatty deposition syndrome" *Adv Skin Wound Care.* 23: 81–92. doi: 10.1097/01.ASW.0000363503.92360.91.

Fioretti, C. vd. (2016). "Research studies on patients' illness experience using the narrative medicine approach: a systematic review" *BMJ Open* 6: e011220. doi: 10.1136/ bmjopen-2016-011220

Florjański, J. vd. (2001). "The course of pregnancy, delivery and puerperium in women with varices and thrombophlebitis of lower extremities, after application of low molecular weight heparins"*Ginekol Pol* 72(12A): 1291–1295

Flour, M., Clark, M., Partsch, H. vd. (2013). "Dogmas and controversies in compression therapy: report of an International Compression Club (ICC) meeting, Brussels, May 2011" Int Wound J 10: 516–526

Foley, E., Matheis, R., Schaefer, C. (2002). "Effect of forced laughter on mood" *Psychol Rep.* 90(1): 184.

Fonseca-Alaniz, M.H., Takada, J., Alonso-Vale, M.I.C., Lima, F.B. (2006). "The adipose tissue as a regulatory center of the metabolism" Arq Bras Endocrinol Metab, 50: 216-229

Ford, A.L. vd. (2010). "Treatment of childhood obesity by retraining eating behaviour: randomised controlled trial" *BMJ* 340: b5388

Forner-Cordero, I., Szolnoky, G., Forner-Cordero, A., Kemeny, L. (2012). "Lipedema: an overview of its clinical manifestations, diagnosis and treatment of the disproportional fatty deposition syndrome - systematic review" *Clin Obes.* 2: 86–95

Földi, E., Földi, M. (2005). "Das Lipödem" *Lehrbuch der Lymphologie für Mediziner, Masseure und Physiotherapeuten.* Munich Elsevier, Urban&Fischer, 443-453.

Földi, M., Földi, E., Kubik, S. (2005). *Textbook of Lymphology*, New York: Elsevier

Freese, J., Klement, R.J., Ruiz-Núñez, B., Schwarz, S., Lötzerich, H. (2017). "The sedentary (r)evolution: Have we lost our metabolic flexibility?" F1000Res. Oct 2;6: 1787

Fried, M., Abramson, S., Meyer, J.H. (1987). "Passage of salivary amylase through the stomach in humans" *Dig. Dis. Sci.* 32: 1097–1103.

Fuss, J., Uhlig, G., Böhme, M. (2018). "Earliest evidence of caries lesion in hominids reveal sugar-rich diet for a Middle Miocene dryopithecine from Europe" *PLoS One.* 13(8):e0203307 doi:10.1371/journal.pone.0203307

Gaby, A. (2013). "A review of the fundamentals of diet" *Glob Adv Health Med.* 2(1):58-63.

Galanaud, J.P, Laroche, J.P., Righini, M. (2013). "The history and historical treatments of deep vein thrombosis" *J Thromb Haemost.* 11(3): 402–411

Garcia Hidalgo, L. (2002). "Dermatological complications of obesity" *Am J Clin Dermatol.* 3:497–506.

Garcia-Martinez, O., Ruiz, C., Gutierrez-Ibanez, A., Illescas-Montes, R., Melguizo-Rodriguez, L. (2018). "Benefits of Olive Oil Phenolic Compounds in Disease Prevention" Endocr. Metab. Immune Disord. Drug Targets. 18:333–340.

Gardner, A.M., Fox, R.H. (1993). "Peripheral venous physiology" In: Gardner AM, Fox RH, editors. The return of the blood to the heart London: John Libbey; 61-87.

Garg, A. (2011). "Clinical review: lipodystrophies: genetic and acquired body fat disorders" *J Clin Endocrinol Metab.* 96(11):3313–3325

Gaskell, P., Parrott, J.C. (1978). "The effect of a mechanical venous pump on the circulation of the feet in the presence of arterial obstruction" *Surg Gynecol Obstet.* 146: 583–592

Gatchel, R.J., Neblett, R. (2022). "Pain catastrophizing: what clinicians need to know" Practical Pain Management. Accessed February 2, 2022

Gauer, R.L. (2011). "Evaluation of syncope" Am. Fam. Physician 84, 640–650

Gazit, Y., Nahir, A.M., Grahame, R., Jacob, G. (2003). "Dysautonomia in the joint hypermobility syndrome" *Am J Med.* 115(1): 33-40

Geloneze, B., Tambascia, M.A. (2006). "Laboratorial evaluation and diagnosis of insulin resistance" Arq Bras Endocrinol Metabol. 50(2): 208–215.

Genoni, A. vd. (2019). "Paleolithic diet lowers resistant starch intake but does not affect serum trimethylamine-N-oxide concentrations in healthy women" *Br. J. Nutr.* 121(3):322-329.

Gerson, R.M. (1997). "Avoiding end hits in ultrasound-assisted lipoplasty" *Aesthetic Surg* J 17:331–332.

Gibson, W.S. (1966). "Hippocrates' home" *JAMA* (197):628–631

Giese, S.Y., Bulan, E.J., Commons, G.W. vd. (2001). "Improvements in cardiovascular risk profile with large-volume liposuction: a pilot study" Plast Reconstr Surg. 108: 510–519; discussion 520

Gill, S.R., Pop, M., Deboy, R.T. vd. (2006). "Metagenomic analysis of the human distal gut microbiome" Science. 312(5778): 1355–1359.

Giugliano, G., Nicoletti, G., Grella, E. vd. (2004). "Effect of liposuction on insulin resistance and vascular inflammatory markers in obese women" Br J Plast Surg. 57:190–194

Glomset, J.A. (1985). "Fish, fatty acids, and human health" N Engl J Med 312: 1253-1254

Gloviczki, P., Comerota, A.J., Dalsing, M.C. vd. (2011). "The care of patients with varicose veins and associated chronic venous diseases: clinical practice guidelines of the Society for Vascular Surgery and the American Venous Forum" *J Vasc Surg* 53(Suppl): 2S–48S

Gloviczki, P., Gloviczki, M.L. (2012). "Guidelines for the management of varicose veins" *Phlebology* 27(Suppl 1): 2–9

Gluckman, P., Hanson, M. (2008). *Mismatch: The Lifestyle Diseases Timebomb*, Oxford University Press, New York

Goldberg, H. (2006). *HIPPOCRATES: Father of Medicine,* iUniverse Press

Goldman, M.P. (2002). "Treatment of varicose and telangiectatic leg veins: double-blind prospective comparative trial between aethoxyskerol and sotradecol" *Dermatologic Surgery* 28(1): 52-55

Goldman, M.P. (2004). "Optimal management of facial telangiectasia" *American Journal of Clinical Dermatology* 5(6): 423-434.

Golparvar, M., Kamkar, M., & Rismanchian, B. (2008). "Investigating relationship of Overweight with self-esteem, depression, lifestyle, and physical self-concept in self-introduced women of weight loss centers" Research in Psychology, 32, 121-144.

Goncharov, I. (2005). *Oblomov,* Penguin Classics

González Carretero, L., Wollstonecroft, M., Fuller, D. Q. (2017). "A methodological approach to the study of archaeological cereal meals: A case study at Çatalhöyük East (Turkey)" *Veg. Hist. Archaeobot.* 26, 415–432

Goodman, A. (1993). "On the Interpretation ofHealth from Skeletal Remains" Current Anthropology, 34(3): 281-288.

Grahame, R. (1992). "A proposed set of diagnostic criteria for the benign joint hypermobility syndrome" *Br J Rheumatol* 31: 205

Grazer, F.M., de Jong, R.H. (2000). "Fatal outcomes from liposuction: census survey of cosmetic surgeons" Plast Reconstr Surg. 105:436–446

Greenhalgh, T., Hurwitz, B. (ed.) (1998). *Narrative based medicine. Dialogue and discourse in clinical practice,* BMJ Books, London.

Greenhalgh, T., Hurwitz, B. (1998). "Why study narrative?" *Narrative based medicine. Dialogue and discourse in clinical practice.* Greenhalgh T, Hurwitz B, editors. London, UK: BMJ Books; 3–16

Greer, K.E. (1974). "Lipedema of the legs" *Cutis* 14: 98.

Gregor, M.F., Hotamisligil, G.S. (2011). "Inflammatory mechanisms in obesity" Annu Rev Immunol 29: 415–445

Grice, E.A. vd. (2009). "Topographical and temporal diversity of the human skin microbiome" Science 324: 1190–1192.

Grice, E.A., Segre, J.A. (2011). "The skin microbiome" Nat Rev Microbiol 9: 244–253.

Grimes, P.E. (2009). "Management of hyperpigmentation in darker racial ethnic groups" *Semin Cutan Med Surg.* 28: 77-85.

Grolleau, J.L., Rouge, D., Chavoin, J.P., Costagliola, M. (1997). "Severe cutaneous necrosis after ultrasound lipolysis. Medicolegal aspects and review" *Ann Chir Plast Esthet* 42:31–36.

Grossbart, T.A, Sarwer, D.B. (1999). "Cosmetic surgery: Surgical tools—Psychosocial goals" *Semin Cutan Med Surg.* 18: 101

Grossman, P., Niemann, L., Schmidt, S., Walach, H. (2004). "Mindfulness-based stress reduction and health benefits: A meta-analysis" *J. Psychosom. Res.* 57:35–43. doi: 10.1016/S0022-3999(03)00573-7

Guebre-Egziabher, F. vd. (2013). "Ectopic lipid accumulation: a potential cause for metabolic disturbances and a contributor to the alteration of kidney function" *Biochimie* 95(11): 1971–1979

Guéguen, N. (2012). "Color and women attractiveness: when red clothed women are perceived to have more intense sexual intent" *J. Soc. Psychol.* 152: 261–265. 10.1080/00224545.2011.605398

Guéguen, N. (2015). "High heels increase women's attractiveness" *Arch. Sex. Behav.* 44: 2227–2235. 10.1007/s10508-014-0422-z

Hainsworth, R. (2004). "Pathophysiology of syncope" Clin Auton Res. 14 Suppl 1: 18–24.

Hardy, K. (2019). "Paleomedicine and the use of plant secondary compounds in the Paleolithic and Early Neolithic" Evol Anthropol. Mar; 28(2): 60-71.

Hagemann, D., Meier, J.J., Gallwitz, B., Schmidt, W.E. (2003). "Appetite regulation by ghrelin – a novel neuro-endocrine gastric peptide hormone in the gut-brain-axis" Z Gastroenterol 41: 929–936

Halk, A.B., Damstra, R.J. (2017). "Firt Dutch guidelines on lipedema using the international classification of functioning, disability and helath" *Phlebology*, 32: 152-159

Hallgren, E. vd. (2015). "Dysfunctional vestibular system causes a blood pressure drop in astronauts returning from space" Sci. Rep. 5, 17627

Halter, J.B., Beard, J.C., Porte, D. (1984). "Jr Islet functions and stress hyperglycemia: Plasma glucose and epinephrine interaction" Am J Physiol. 247: E47–52.

Hamel-Desnos, C.M., Guias, B.J., Desnos, P.R. vd. (2010). "Foam sclerotherapy of the saphenous veins: randomised controlled trial with or without compression" *Eur J Vasc Endovasc Surg* 39: 500–507

Hardy, D. vd. (2017). "Best Practice Guidelines: The management of lipoedema" Wounds UK vol.13, London http://www.wounds-uk.com/best-practice-statements/best-practice-guidelines-the-management-of-lipoedema.

Harvey, N.L. vd. (2005). "Lymphatic vascular defects promoted by Prox1 haploinsufficiency cause adult-onset obesity" *Nat Genet* 37: 1072-1081.

Harwood, C.A. vd. (1996). "Lymphatic and venous function in lipoedema" *Br J Dermatol.* 134: 16.

Hassan, A., Tooke, J. (1988). "Effect of changes in local skin temper- ature on postural vasoconstriction in man" *Clin Sci* 74: 201–206.

Hassan, A., Carter, G., Tooke, J. (1990). "Postural vasoconstriction in women during the normal menstrual cycle" *Clin Sci* 78: 39–47.

Hayden, B. (2012). "Corporate Groups and Secret Societies in the Early Neolithic. A Comment on Hodder and Meskell" Current Anthropology 53, 1, 126-127.

Herbst, K.L. (2012). "Rare adipose disorders (RADs) masquerading as obesity" *Acta Pharmacol Sin* 33: 155-172.

Herbst, K., Mirkovskaya, L., Bharhagava, A., Chava, Y., Te, C.H. (2015). "Lipedema fat and signs and symptoms of illness, increase with advancing stage" *Archieves of medicine*, vol.7 no: 4:10, 1–8

Herbst, K.L. (2019). "Subcutaneous Adipose Tissue Diseases: Dercum Disease, Lipedema, Familial Multiple Lipomatosis, and Madelung Disease" *Endotext [Internet].* South Dartmouth (MA): MDText.com.

Herpertz, U. (2004). "Ödeme und Lymphdrainage. Diagnose und Therapie von Ödemkrankheiten 2nd edition" *Schattauer*, Stuttgart New York 168-181.

Herrero, S. (2003). *Bear Attacks: Their Causes and Avoidance, New Revised Edition.* Toronto: McClelland and Stewart Ltd

Hernandez, T.L. vd. (2011). "Fat redistri- bution following suction lipectomy: defense of body fat and patterns of restoration" *Obesity (Silver Spring)* 19:1388–1395

Hetherington, M.M., Cecil, J.E. (2010). "Gene-environment interactions in obesity" *Forum Nutr.* 63: 195-203. doi: 10.1159/000264407. Epub 2009 Nov 27.

Hewlings, S.J., Kalman, D.S. (2017). "Curcumin: A Review of Its Effects on Human Health" Foods. 6(10): 92

Hirai, M. vd. (2008). "Interface pressure and stiffness of various elastic stockings during posture changes and exercise" *Vascular* 16: 9– 100.

Hirosaki, M. vd. (2013). "Effects of a laughter and exercise program on physiological and psychological health among community-dwelling elderly in Japan: Randomized controlled trial" *Geriatr Gerontol Int,* 13(1), 152–160. 10.1111/j.1447-0594.2012.00877.x

Holick, M.F. (1999)."Vitamin D" In: *Modern nutrition in health and disease.* Shils M.E., Olson J.A., Shike M., Ross A.C., editors. Lippincott; Williams & Wilkins: 228–239.

Holick, M.F., Chen, T.C. (2008). "Vitamin D deficiency: A worldwide problem with health consequences" Am J Clin Nutr. 87: 1080S–6S.

Holland, K.T., Bojar, R.A. (2002). "Cosmetics: what is their influence on the skin microflora?" Am J Clin Dermatol 3: 445–449

Holowka, N.B., Wallace, I.J., Lieberman, D.E. (2018). "Foot strength and stiffness are related to footwear use in a comparison of minimally- vs. conventionally-shod populations" Sci Rep. Feb 27; 8(1): 3679.

Holscher, H.D. vd. (2018). "Walnut Consumption Alters the Gastrointestinal Microbiota,

Microbially Derived Secondary Bile Acids, and Health Markers in Healthy Adults: A Randomized Controlled Trial" The Journal of Nutrition, Volume 148, Issue 6, June, 861–867

Hong, S.M., Ko, J.K., Moon, J.J., Kim, Y.R. (2021). "Oxytocin: A Potential Therapeutic for Obesity" J Obes Metab Syndr. Jun 30; 30(2): 115-123.

Horwitz, C., Walker, A.R.P. (1984). "Lignans—additional benefits from fiber?" *Nutr Cancer* 6: 73–76

Housman, T.S, Lawrence, N., Mellen, B.G. vd. (2002). "The safety of liposuction: results of a national survey" Dermatol Surg. 28: 971–978

Howard, B.K., Beran, S.J., Kenkel, J.M., Krueger, J., Rohrich, R.J. (1999). "The effects of ultrasonic energy on peripheral nerves: implications for ultrasound-assisted liposuction" *Plast Reconstr Surg* 103:984–989.

Ignaciuk, A. (2004). "Diagnostyka kliniczna – cellulite" *Mag Med Estet.* 1: 15–7

Ilizarov, S., Rozbruch, S. R. (2007). "Limb Lengthening and Reconstruction Surgery" New York: Informa Healthcare USA Inc.675–679.

Ito, E., Shima, R., Yoshioka, T. (2019). "A novel role of oxytocin: Oxytocin-induced well-being in humans" Biophys Physicobiol. Aug 24; 16: 132-139.

Jagtman, B.A., Kuiper, J.P., Brakkee, A.J. (1984) "Measurments of skin elasticity in patients with lipoedema of the moncorps 'rusticanus' type" *Phlebologie* 37(3): 315–319

Janda, K., Tomikowska, A. (2014). "Cellulit - przyczyny, profilaktyka, leczenie (Cellulite - causes, prevention, treatment)" *Ann Acad Med Stetin.* 60(1):29-38.

Janiak, M.C. (2016). "Digestive enzymes of human and nonhuman primates" *Evolutionary Anthropology: Issues, News, and Reviews.* 25:253–266

Jastroch, M., Seebacher, F. (2020). "Importance of adipocyte browning in the evolution of endothermy" Philos Trans R Soc Lond B Biol Sci. Mar 2; 375(1793): 20190134.

Jäpelt, R.B., Jakobsen. J. (2013). "Vitamin D in plants: a review of occurrence, analysis, and biosynthesis" Front Plant Sci. May 13; 4: 136.

Jeffery, R.W., Epstein, L.H., Wilson, G.T., Drewnowski, A. (2000). "Long-term maintenance of weight loss: current status" *Health Psychol* 19: 5–16

Jensen, M.D., Kanaley, J.A., Reed, J.E., Sheedy, P.F. (1995). "Measurement of abdominal and visceral fat with computed tomography and dual-energy x-ray absorptiometry" Am J Clin Nutr 61:274–278

Kabat-Zinn, J., Davidson, R.J. (2011). "The mind's own physician: A scientific dialogue with the Dalai Lama on the healing power of meditation" Oakland, CA: New Harbinger

Kahn, S.R., Shapiro, S., Wells, P.S. vd. (2014). "Compression stockings to prevent post-thrombotic syndrome: a randomised placebo-controlled trial" *Lancet* 383: 880–888.

Kaiserling, E. (2006). "Morphological changes in lymphedema and tumors," *Földi's Textbook of Lymphology*, M. Földi and E. Földi, Eds., 321–390, Elsevier GmbH, Munich, Germany

Kalitzkus, V., Matthiessen, P.F. (2009). "Narrative-based medicine: potential, pitfalls and practice" *Perm J.* 13(1): 80–86

Kaoutzanis, C. vd. (2017). "Cosmetic Liposuction: Preoperative Risk Factors, Major Complication Rates, and Safety of Combined Procedures" *Aesthet Surg J.* Jun 1;37(6): 680-694. doi: 10.1093/asj/sjw243.

Kaplan, H. vd. (2017). "Coronary atherosclerosis in indigenous South American Tsimane: a cross-sectional cohort study" Lancet. 389(10080): 1730–1739.

Karkkainen, M.J., Saaristo, A., Jussila, L. vd. (2001). "A model for gene therapy of human hereditary lymphedema" *Proc Natl Acad Sci U S A* 98: 12677-12682

Kasper, D.L. vd. (2005). *Harrison's Principles of Internal Medicine. 16th ed* McGraw-Hill,

New York

Kasperczak, J., Ropacka-Lesiak, M., Breborowicz, H.G. (2013). "Definition, classification and diagnosis of chronic venous insufficiency - part II" *Ginekol Pol.* 84(1): 51–55

Kawai, M., de Paula, F.J., Rosen, C.J. (2012). "New insights into osteoporosis: the bone-fat connection" *J Intern Med.* 272(4): 317–329

Kennedy, G.C. (1953). "The role of depot fat in the hypothalamic control of food intake in the rat" Proc R Soc Lond B Biol Sci. 140(901): 578–596.

Kennedy, G.C. (1957). "The development with age of hypothalamic restraint upon the appetite of the rat" J Endocrinol 16: 9–17.

Kershaw, E., Flier, J. (2004). "Adipose tissue as an endocrine organ" *J Clin Endocrinol Metab* 89: 2548–2556

Khoury, B. vd. (2013). "Mindfulness-based therapy: A comprehensive meta-analysis" *Clin. Psychol. Rev.* 33: 763–771. doi: 10.1016/j.cpr.2013.05.005

Killingsworth, M.A., Gilbert, D.T. (2010). "A Wandering Mind is an Unhappy Mind" Science. 330: 1-6. Doi: 10.1126/science

Kissebah, A.H., Krakower, G.R. (1994). "Regional adiposity and morbidity" *Physiol Rev* 74: 761–811

Klassen, A., Jenkinson, C., Fitzpatrick, R., Goodacre, T. (1996). "Patients' health related quality of life before and after aesthetic surgery" *Br J Plast Surg.* Oct; 49(7): 433-438.

Knechtle, B., Waśkiewicz, Z., Sousa, C.V., Hill, L. Nikolaidis, P.T. (2020). "Cold Water Swimming—Benefits and Risks: A Narrative Review" Int J Environ Res Public Health. Dec; 17(23): 8984.

Kobal, D., Musek, J. (2001). "Self-concept and academic achievement: Slovenia and France" Personality and Individual Differences, 30, 887-899.

Kozel, B.A., Danback, J.R., Waxler, J.L. vd. (2014). "Williams syndrome predisposes to vascular stiffness modified by antihypertensive use and copy number changes in NCF1" Hypertension 63:74-79.

Krijnen, R.M.A., De Boer, E.M., Ader, H.J., Bruynzeel, D.P. (1999). "Venous insufficiency in male workers with a standing profession: Epidemiology and prevention" ANZ J Phleb 3: 4-12

Kröger, K. vd. (2017). "Verordnungslogik von medizinischen Kompressionstrümpfen bei Patienten mit chronischer venöser Insuffizienz" *Vasomed* 29: 199– 201.

Krylov, I.A. (2012). *Krilof and His Fables*, Hard Press Publishing

Kuiper, N.A., Martin, R.A. (1998). "Laughter and stress in daily life: relation to positive and negative affect" *Motiv Emot.* 22: 133-153

Kuzma, J.N. vd. (2019). "Intraindividual Variation in Markers of Intestinal Permeability and Adipose Tissue Inflammation in Healthy Normal-Weight to Obese Adults" *Cancer Epidemiol Biomarkers Prev.* 28(3): 610–615. 10.1158/1055-9965.EPI-18-0641

Lamont, R.J., Koo, H., Hajishengallis, G. (2018). "The oral microbiota: dynamic communities and host interactions" Nat. Rev. Microbiol., 16 (12): 745-759

Lang, C., Peters, J., Pöllath, N., Schmidt, K., Grupe, G. (2013). "Gazelle behavior and human presence at early Neolithic Göbekli Tepe, SE Anatolia" Journal of World Archaeology 45, 3, 410-429.

Langendoen, S.I., Habbema, L., Nijsten, T.E.C., Neumann, H.A.M. (2009). "Lipoedema: from clinical presentation to therapy. A review of the literature" Br J Dermatol. 161(5): 980–986.

Larbey, C., Mentzer, S.M., Ligouis, B., Wurz, S., Jones, M.K. (2019). "Cooked starchy food in hearths ca. 120 kya and 65 kya (MIS 5e and MIS 4) from Klasies River Cave, South

Africa" *Journal of Human Evolution.* 131:210–227.

Larsen, C.S. (1981). "Skeletal and Dental Adaptations to the Shift to Agriculture on the Georgia Coast". Current Anthropology, 22(4): 422-423.

Larsen, C.S. (2006). "The Agricultural Revolution as Environmental Catastrophe: Implications for Health and Lifestyle in the Holocene" Quaternary International, 150(1): 12-20.

Larsen, T.M. vd. (2010). "Diets with high or low protein content and glycemic index for weight-loss maintenance" *N Engl J Med* 363: 2102-2113

Lassek, W. D., Gaulin, S. J. (2006). "Changes in body fat distribution in relation to parity in American women: a covert form of maternal depletion" *Am. J. Phys. Anthropol.* 131, 295–302

Lassek W. D., Gaulin S. J. (2007). "Waist-hip ratio and cognitive ability: is gluteofemoral fat a privileged store of neurodevelopmental resources?" *Evol. Hum. Behav.* 29, 26–34

Launer, J. (2002). Narrative-based Primary Care: A practical guide (1st ed.). CRC Press. https://doi.org/10.1201/9781315385549

Launer J. (2013). "Training in narrative-based supervision: conversations inviting change" *Clinical uncertainty in primary care. The challenge of collaborative engagement.* Sommers L.S ve Launer J. (ed.) New York, NY: Springer; 163–176

Launer, J. (2018). "John Launer on narrative based medicine" Available from: www.gp-training.net/training/communication_skills/consultation/narrative_launer.htm. Accessed 2018 Jan 23

Lazaridis, I. vd. (2014). "Ancient human genomes suggest three ancestral populations for present-day Europeans" Nature. Sep 18; 513(7518): 409-13

Le Hénaff, Y. (2017). "Cosmetic Surgery on Trial: How the Dujarier Case Impacted its Practice and Structure in France during the Interwar Period" *Social History of Medicine*, Oxford University Press (OUP), 10.1093/shm/hkx054 hal-01684141

Lee, R., Kean, W.F. (2012). "Obesity and knee osteoarthritis" Inflammopharmacology. Apr; 20(2): 53-58.

Leszko, M. (2014). "Cellulite in menopause" *Prz Menopauzalny* 13(5): 298–304

Levi, M. (2005). "Vasovagal fainting as an evolutionary remnant of the fight against hemorrhage" Clin Auton Res 15, 69–70

Lewis, B. (2011). "Narrative and psychiatry" *Curr Opin Psychiatry* 24(6): 489–494

Ley, R.E., Peterson, D.A., Gordon, J.I. (2006). "Ecological and evolutionary forces shaping microbial diversity in the human intestine" Cell. 124(4): 837–848

Ley, R.E., Turnbaugh, P.J., Klein, S., Gordon, J.I. (2006). "Microbial ecology: Human gut microbes associated with obesity" *Nature* 444: 1022–1023

Li, H. vd. (2011). "Adipogenic potential of adipose stem cell subpopulations" *Plast Reconstr Surg* 128: 663-672.

Lim, C.S., Davies, A.H. (2014). "Graduated compression stockings" *CMAJ* 186(10): 391-398 doi:101503/cmaj.131281

Lin, S.K. (2001). "The Nature of the Chemical Process. 1. Symmetry Evolution—Revised Information Theory, Similarity Principle and Ugly Symmetry" *Int. J. Mol. Sci.* 2, 10–39.

Little, T.J., Horowitz, M., Feinle-Bisset, C. (2005). "Role of cholecystokinin in appetite control and body weight regulation" Obes Rev 6:297–306

Lobionda, S., Sittipo, P., Kwon, H.Y., Lee, Y.K. (2019). "The role of gut microbiota in intestinal inflammation with respect to diet and extrinsic stressors" Microorganisms. 7: 271. doi: 10.3390/microorganisms7080271

Lohrmann, C., Foeldi, E., Langer, M. (2009). "MR imaging of the lymphatic system in patients with lipedema and lipo-lymphedema" *Microvasc Res.* 77: 335–339

Longo, V.D., Panda, S. (2016). "Fasting, circadian rhythms, and time restricted feeding in healthy lifespan" Cell Metab. Jun 14; 23(6): 1048–1059. DOI: 10.1016/j.cmet.2016.06.001

Lowe, M.R. (2003). "Self regulation of energy intake in the prevention and treatment of obesity: is it feasible?" *Obes Res* 11: 44–59

Ludwig, D.S. (2002). "The glycemic index: physiological mechanisms relating to obesity, diabetes, and cardiovascular disease" *JAMA* 287:2414-23. 10.1001/jama.287.18.2414

Ludwig, D.S., Friedman, M.I. (2014). "Increasing adiposity: consequence or cause of overeating?" *JAMA* 311:2167-2168. 10.1001/jama.2014.4133

Ludwig, D.S., Ebbeling, C.B. (2018). "The Carbohydrate-Insulin Model of Obesity: Beyond 'Calories In, Calories Out'" *JAMA Intern Med* 178:1098-103. 10.1001/jamainternmed.2018.2933

Lupi, O., Semenovitch, I., Treu, C. vd. (2007). "Evaluation of the effects of caffeine in the microcirculation and edema on thighs and buttocks using the orthogonal polarization spectral imaging and clinical parameters" *J Cosmet Dermatol* 6: 102–107

Lykkesfeldt, J., Michels, A.J., Frei, B. (2014). "Vitamin C" Adv Nutr. Jan 1; 5(1): 16-18.

Lykkesfeldt, J. (2020). "On the effect of vitamin C intake on human health: How to (mis) interprete the clinical evidence" Redox Biol. Jul; 34: 101532

Macgregor, G.A., Markandu, N.D., Roulston, J.E., Jones, J.C., de Wardemer, H.E. (1979). "Is 'idiopathic' oedema idiopathic?" *Lancet* i:397–400.

Majzoub, J.A. (2006). "Corticotropin-releasing hormone physiology" European Journal of Endocrinology. 155(suppl 1): 71–76.

Mailer, G. (2015). "Decolonizing the Diet: synthesizing Native- American history, immunology, and nutritional science" Journal of Evolution and Health An Ancestral Health Society Publication 1 (1)

Malhotra, S.L. (1972). "An epidemiological study of varicose veins in Indian railroad workers from the south and north of India, with special reference to the causation and prevention of varicose veins" Int J Epidemiol 1: 177-183.

Mallon, E., Powell, S., Mortimer, P., Ryan, T.J. (1997). "Evidence for altered cell-mediated immunity in postmastectomy lymphedema" Br J Dermatol. 137:928–933. doi: 10.1111/j.1365-2133.1997.tb01553.x.

Maltz, M. (2015). *Psycho-Cybernetics: Updated And Expanded*, TarcherPerigee, an imprint of Penguin Random House LLC

Manheimer, E.W., van Zuuren, E.J., Fedorowicz, Z., Pijl, H. (2015). "Paleolithic nutrition for metabolic syndrome: systematic review and meta-analysis" Am J Clin Nutr. Oct;102(4): 922-32

Manolopoulos, K.N., Karpe, F., Frayn, K.N. (2010). "Gluteofemoral body fat as a determinant of metabolic health" *Int J Obes (Lond).* Jun; 34(6):949-59. doi: 10.1038/ijo.2009.286.

Mantzios, M., Wilson, J.C. (2015). "Mindfulness, eating behaviours, and obesity: a review and reflection on current findings" *Curr. Obes. Rep.* 4:141–146. doi: 10.1007/s13679-014-0131-x

Mariani, F., Marone, E.M., Gasbarro, V. vd. (2011). "Multicenter randomized trial comparing compression with elastic stocking versus bandage after surgery for varicose veins" *J Vasc Surg* 53: 115–122

Marks, I.M., Nesse, R.M. (1994). "Fear and fitness: an evolutionary analysis of anxiety disorders" *Ethol Sociobiol* 15: 247-261

Marque, M., Girard, C., Guillot, B., Bessis, D. (2008). "Superfi- cial lymphangitis after arthropod bite: a distinctive but underrecognized entity?" Dermatology 217: 262–267.

Marsch, W.C. (2001). "Ist das Lipödem ein lymphologisches Kranheitsbild?" *J Lymphologie* 1: 22-24

Marshall, M., Schwahn-Schreiber, C. (2011). "Prevalence of lipoedema in professional women in Germany" *Phlebologie* 40: 127-134.

Martarelli, D., Cocchioni, M., Scuri, S., Pompei, P. (2011). "Diaphragmatic breathing reduces exercise-induced oxidative stress" Evid. Based Complement. Altern. Med. 2011:932430. doi: 10.1093/ecam/nep169

Martin, S., Edward, M.C., Peter, C. (2005). "Lymph makes you fat" *Nature Genetics*. 37(10): 1023

Masterson, M., Morgan, A. (2006). "The Role of Lower Leg Muscle Activity in Blood Pressure Maintenance of Older Adults" *Clin. Kinesiol.* 60, 8–18

Mathews, W.A., Grazer, F.M. (1992). "Operative management. Atlas of Suction Assisted Lipectomy in Body Contouring" New York, Churchill Livingstone; 69–98

Mathur, N., Pedersen, B.K. (2008). "Exercise as a mean to control low-grade systemic inflammation" *Mediators of Inflammation* vol. 2008, Article ID 109502, 6 pages, 2008. https://doi.org/10.1155/2008/109502

Matthews, CM. (2012). "Exploring the obesity epidemic" Proc (Bayl Univ Med Cent). Jul; 25(3): 276-277.

Mattson, M.P. (2019). "An Evolutionary Perspective on Why Food Overconsumption Impairs Cognition Trends" Cogn Sci. Mar; 23(3): 200–212.

Mauer, M.M., Harris, R.B., Bartness, T.J. (2001). "The regulation of total body fat: lessons learned from lipectomy studies" Neurosci Biobehav Rev. 25(1): 15–28.

Mayes, J.S., Watson, G.H. (2004). "Direct effects of sex steroid hormones on adipose tissues and obesity" Obes Rev 5:197-216.

Medina-Gómez, G. (2012). "Mitochondria and endocrine function of adipose tissue" *Best Pract Res Clin Endocrinol Metab.* 26(6):791–804.

Meier-Vollrath, I., Schmeller, W. (2004). "Lipoedema: current status, new perspectives" *J Dtsch Dermatol Ges.* 2:181–186.

Mekki, N., Christofilis, M.A., Charbonnier, M. vd. (1999). "Influence of obesity and body fat distribution on postprandial lipemia and triglyceride-rich lipoproteins in adult women" *J Clin Endocrinol Metab* 84: 184-191.

Mekky, S., Schilling, R.S.F., Walford, J. (1969). "Varicose veins in English cotton workers. An epidemiological study in England and Egypt" Br Med J 2: 591-595.

Meller, C., Urzua, I., Moncada, G., Von Ohle, C. (2009). "Prevalence of Oral Pathologic Findings in an Ancient pre- Columbian Archeological Site in the Atacama Desert" Oral Diseases, 15(4): 287-294.

Mellor, A., Soni, N. (2001). "Fat embolism" Anaesthesia. 56:145–154

Merlen, J.F., Curri, S.B., Sarteel, A.M. (1979). "Cellulitis, a conjunctive microvascular disease" *Phlebologie* 32: 279-282.

Messier, V. vd. (2010). "Identifying metabolically healthy but obese individuals in sedentary postmenopausal women" *Obesity (Silver Spring)* 18(5): 911–917

Metges, C.C. (2000). "Contribution of microbial amino acids to amino acid homeostasis of the host" J Nutr. 130(7): 1857S–64S.

Metges, C.C., Petzke, K.J. (2005). "Utilization of essential amino acids synthesized in the intestinal microbiota of monogastric mammals" Br J Nutr. 94(5): 621–2.

McLean, K.C., Pasupathi, M., (ed.) (2010). *Narrative development in adolescence. Creating the storied self.* New York, Springer

Michl, L.C., McLaughlin, K.A., Shepherd, K., Nolen-Hoeksema, S. (2013). "Rumination as a mechanism linking stressful life events to symptoms of depression and anxiety: longitudinal evidence in early adolescents and adults" J Abnorm Psychol. May;122(2):339-52. doi: 10.1037/a0031994.

Micke, O., vd. (2000). "Selenium in the treatment of acute and chronic lymphedema" *Trace Elements and Electrolytes* 17:206–209.

Mika, A. vd. (2011). "Changes of bioelectrical activity in cervical paraspinal muscle during gait in low and high heel shoes" *Acta Bioeng Biomech*, 13: 27–33.

Minihane, A.M. vd. (2015). "Low-grade inflammation, diet composition and health: current research evidence and its translation" Br J Nutr. Oct 14; 114(7): 999-1012.

Mira, A., Pushker, R., Rodríguez-Valera, F. (2006). "The Neolithic revolution of bacterial genomes" Trends Microbiol. 14: 200–206.

Mogilevskii, I.L., Osmolovskaia, N.N., Deputovich, S.A. (1989). "Microcirculatory disorders of the arm in post-mastectomy edema" *Sov Med.* 15–20

Moncorps, C., Brinkhaus, G., Herfeld-Munster, F. (1940). "Experimental investigations in acrocyanosis" *Arch Dermatol Syph* 180: 209–215

Morin, E. vd. (2019). "New evidence of broader diets for archaic Homo populations in the northwestern Mediterranean" Sci Adv. Mar; 5(3)

Morita, H., Abe, C., Tanaka, K. (2016). "Long-term exposure to microgravity impairs vestibulo-cardiovascular reflex" Sci. Rep. 6, 33405

Morris, D. (1981). *The Soccer Tribe,* 1st edition, London: Jonathan Cape.

Morris, J.N., Hardman, A.E. (1997). "Walking to health" Sports Med. May; 23(5): 306-332.

Morris, P.H., White, J., Morrison, E.R., Fisher, K. (2013). "High heels as supernormal stimuli: how wearing high heels affects judgements of female attractiveness" *Evol. Hum. Behav.* 34: 176–181. 10.1016/j.evolhumbehav.2012.11.006

Mortimer, P.S. (1995). "Managing lymphedema" Clin Dermatol. 13:499–505.

Mortimer, P.S., Levick, J.R. (2004). "Chronic peripheral oedema: the critical role of the lymphatic system" Clin Med (Lond). 4(5): 448-453. doi:10.7861/clinmedicine.4-5-448

Motykie, G.D., Caprini, J.A., Arcelus, J.I. vd. (1999). "Evaluation of therapeutic compression stockings in the treatment of chronic venous insufficiency" *Dermatol Surg* 25: 116–120

Moura, V., Monteiro, R. (2010). "Papel do tecido adiposo na inflamação e metabolismo do doente obeso" Revista da SPCNA, 16. 15-22

Mousa, H.A. (2016). "Health Effects of Alkaline Diet and Water, Reduction of Digestive-tract Bacterial Load, and Earthing" Altern Ther Health Med. Apr; 22 Suppl 1: 24-33. PMID: 27089527.

Mueller, S.O. vd. (2004). "Phytoestrogens and their human metabolites show distinct agonistic and antagonistic properties on estrogen receptor α (ERα) and ERβ in human cells" Toxicol. Sci. 80: 14-25View in Article Scopus (356)

Murakami, K., Miyake, Y., Sasaki, S., Tanaka K., Arakawa, M. (2012). "Self-reported rate of eating and risk of overweight in Japanese children: Ryukyus child health study" *J. Nutr. Sci. Vitaminol.* 58(4):247–252

Muthuchamy, M., Zawieja, D. (2008). "Molecular regulation of lymphatic contractility" *Ann N Y Acad Sci.* 1131: 89–99

Nagle, D.B., Burstein, S.M. (2002). "The Ancient World: Readings in Social and Cultural History" Prentice Hall, 354

Naidu, K.A. (2003). "Vitamin C in human health and disease is still a mystery? An overview"

Nutr J. Aug 21; 2: 7. doi: 10.1186/1475-2891-2-7.

Nair, R., Maseeh, A. (2012). "Vitamin D: The 'sunshine' vitamin" J Pharmacol Pharmacother. Apr; 3(2): 118-26.

Nakatsuji, T. vd. (2017). "Antimicrobials from human skin commensal bacteria protect against Staphylococcus aureus and are deficient in atopic dermatitis" Sci Transl Med 9

Naouri, M. vd. (2010). "High-resolution cutaneous ultrasonography to differentiate lipoedema from lymphedema" *Br J Dermatol.* Aug;163(2):296-301. doi: 10.1111/j.1365-2133.2010.09810.x. Epub 2010 Apr 16

Narvaez, D., Valentino, K., Fuentes, A., McKenna, J.J., Gray, P. (2014). *Ancestral Landscapes in Human Evolution: Culture, Childrearing and Social Wellbeing,* Oxford University Press, New York

Neel, J.V. (1999). "The 'thrifty genotype' in 1998" Nutrition Reviews. 57: 2–9

Neel, V. (1962). "Diabetes mellitus: a 'thrifty' genotype rendered detrimental by 'progress'?" *Am. J. Hum. Genet.* 14, 353–362

Nelson, J.B. (2017). "Mindful Eating: The Art of Presence While You Eat" *Diabetes Spectr* 30(3):171-174.

Nesse, R.M., Williams, G.C. (1994). *Why We Get Sick: The New Science of Darwinian Medicine*, Vintage, New York.

Nesse, R.M., Williams, G.C. (1999). "Research designs that address evolutionary questions about medical disorders" Stearns SC, ed. *Evolution in Health and Disease*. New York, NY: Oxford University Press; 16-26.

Nesse, R.M., Stearns, S.C. (2008). "The great opportunity: evolutionary applications to medicine and public health" Evolutionary Applications. 1:28–48.

Neto, M.S, da Silva, A.L., Lemos, A., Garcia, B., Marcia, F. (2007). "Quality of life and self-esteem after breast asymmetry surgery" Aesthetic Surgery Journal, 27(6), 616-621.

Neumann, H.A., Partsch, H., Mosti, G., Flour, M. (2016). "Classification of compression stockings: report of the meeting of the International Compression Club, Copenhagen" *Int Angiol* 35: 122–128

Nicolaides A. N. (1997). Investigation of chronic venous insufficiency: A consensus statement (France, March 5-9) Circulation 200010220E126–E163.

Nikitin, A.G. vd. (2019). "Interactions between earliest Linearbandkeramik farmers and central European hunter gatherers at the dawn of European Neolithization" Sci Rep. Dec 20;9(1): 19544

Noël, S. (2014). Cosmetic Surgery, Feminism and Beauty in Early Twentieth-Century France (History of Medicine in Context) 1st Edition, Routledge

Noreik M. vd. (2014). "Resting energy expenditure (REE) in an old-old population: Implications for metabolic stress" *Exp. Gerontol.* 59:47–50.

O'Dea, K. (1991). "Traditional diet and food preferences of Australian aboriginal hunter-gatherers" *Philos Trans R Soc Lond B Biol Sci* 334: 233–241.

O'Dea K. (1997). "Clinical implications of the "thrifty genotype" hypothesis: where do we stand now?" *Nutr Metab Cardiovasc Dis* 7:281–284

Ohlsson, B., Orho-Melander, M., Nilsson, P.M. (2017). "Higher Levels of Serum Zonulin May Rather Be Associated with Increased Risk of Obesity and Hyperlipidemia, Than with Gastrointestinal Symptoms or Disease Manifestations" *Int J Mol Sci.* 18(3): 582. doi:10.3390/ijms18030582

Olde Nordkamp L.R. vd. (2009). Syncope prevalence in the ED compared to general practice and population: a strong selection process. Am J Emerg Med. Mar;27(3):271-9

Oppezzo, M., Schwartz, D.L. (2014). "Give your ideas some legs: the positive effect of walking on creative thinking" J Exp Psychol Learn Mem Cogn. Jul; 40(4): 1142-1152.

Ortonne, J.P., Bissett, D.L. (2008). "Latest insights into skin hyperpigmentation" *J Investig Dermatol Symp Proc.* 13: 10-14

Ottaviani, E. vd. (2011). "Gut microbiota as a candidate for lifespan extension: an ecological/ evolutionary perspective targeted on living organisms as metaorganisms" *Biogerontology* 12 599–609 10.1007/s10522-011-9352-5

Owyang, C., Heldsinger, A. (2011). "Vagal control of satiety and hormonal regulation of appetite" J Neurogastroenterol Motil 17:338–348

Pantano, D. vd. (2016). "Oleuropein aglycone and polyphenols from olive mill wastewater ameliorate cognitive deficits and neuropathology" Br. J. Clin. Pharmacol. https://doi.org/10.1111/bcp.12993

Papathanasiou, A. (2005) "Health Status of the Neolithic Population of Alepotrypa Cave, Greece" American Journal o fPhysical Anthropology, 126:377-390.

Paragliola, R.M. vd. (2021). "Cortisol circadian rhythm and jet-lag syndrome: evaluation of salivary cortisol rhythm in a group of eastward travelers" *Endocrine* 73(2): 424-430

Partsch, H., Stoberl, C., Urbanek, A., Wenzel-Hora, B.I. (1988). "Clinical use of indirect lymphography in different forms of leg edema" *Lymphology*. 21: 152–160

Partsch, H. vd. (1988). "Clinical use of indirect lymphography in different forms of leg edema" *Lymphology* 21: 152-160

Partsch, H., Winiger, N.J., Lun, B. (2004). "Compression stockings reduce occupational leg swelling" Derm Surg. 30: 737-743

Pavlov, V.A., Tracey, K.J. (2012). "The vagus nerve and the inflammatory reflex – linking immunity and metabolism" Nat Rev Endocrinol 8:743–754

Pedersen, B.K. vd. (2003). "Searching for the exercise factor: is IL-6 a candidate?" Journal of Muscle Research and Cell Motility 24(2-3) Vol. 3: 113-119

Pedersen, B.K., Saltin, B. (2006). "Evidence for prescribing exercise as therapy in chronic disease" *Scandinavian Journal of Medicine and Science in Sports* 16: 3-63.

Pedersen, B.K. (2007). "State of the Art Reviews: Health Benefits Related to Exercise in Patients With Chronic Low-Grade Systemic Inflammation" *American Journal of Lifestyle Medicine* 1: 289-298.

Perez, J.A. (1999). "Treatment of dysesthesias secondary to ultrasonic lipoplas-ty" *Plast Reconstr Surg* 103: 1534.

Petersen, A.M.W., Pedersen, B.K. (2005). "The anti-inflammatory effect of exercise" *Journal of Applied Physiology* 98: 1154-1162.

Peterson, J. vd. (2009). "The NIH human microbiome project" Genome Res 19: 2317–2323.

Petrini, L., Arendt-Nielsen, L. (2020). "Understanding Pain Catastrophizing: Putting Pieces Together" Front Psychol. Dec 16; 11: 603420

Pinnick, K.E., Nicholson, G., Manolopoulos, K.N. vd. (2014). "Distinct developmental profile of lower-body adipose tissue defines resistance against obesity-associated metabolic complications" *Diabetes* 63: 3785-3797.

Pirozzi, G. vd. (2013). "Syncope in the elderly: An update" J. Clin. Gerontol. Geriatr. 4, 69–74

Pitt, C.E. (2016). "Cutting through the Paleo hype: The evidence for the Palaeolithic diet" Aust Fam Physician. Jan-Feb; 45(1): 35-8. PMID: 27051985.

Piuri, G. vd. (2021). "Magnesium in Obesity, Metabolic Syndrome, and Type 2 Diabetes" Nutrients. Jan 22; 13(2): 320.

Pollitt, E., Leibel, R.L., Greenfield, D. (1981). "Brief fasting, stress, and cognition in children"

*Am J Clin Nutr.* 34: 1526–1533

Pontzer, H. (2015). "Constrained Total Energy Expenditure and the Evolutionary Biology of Energy Balance" Exerc Sport Sci Rev. Jul; 43(3): 110-116

Porter, J.M., Moneta, G.L. (1995). "Reporting standards in venous disease: an update. International Consensus Committee on Chronic Venous Disease" *Journal of Vascular Surgery* 21(4):635-645

Potter, S.R. (2004). "Commoners, Tribute, and Chiefs: The Development of Algonquian Culture in the Potomac Valley" Charlottesville, 101

Poulos, S., Hausman, D., Hausman, G. (2010). "The development and endocrine functions of adipose tissue" *Mol Cell Endocrinol* 323: 20–34

Pourazizi, M., Kabiri, S., Saffaei, A., Abtahi-Naeini, B. /2017). "Lupus and lupoid misnomer: issues and challenges" Lupus. Jan; 26(1): 6-9.

Pouwels, S., Huisman, S., Smelt, H.J.M., Said, M., Smulders, J.F. (2018). "Lipoedema in patients after bariatric surgery: report of two cases and review of literature" *Clinical Obesity,* vol. 8, no. 2, 147–150

Priglinger, E. vd. (2017). "The adipose tissue-derived stromal vascular fraction cells from lipedema patients: are they different?" *Cytotherapy,* vol. 19, no. 7, 849–860

Prins, J.B. (2002). "Adipose tissue as an endocrine organ" *Best Pract Res Clin Endocrinol Metab* 16: 639–651

Pruzinsky, T., Edgerton, M.T. (1990). "Body-image change in cosmetic plastic surgery" *Body Images: Development, Deviance, and Changes.* Cash TF, Pruzinsky T, editors.New York: Guilford; 217–236

Pruzinsky, T. (1993). "Psychological factors in cosmetic plastic surgery: Recent developments in patient care" *Plast Surg Nurs.* 13:64

Quirke, M. vd. (2017). "Risk factors for nonpurulent leg cellulitis: a systematic review and meta-analysis" Br J Dermatol 177(2): 382-394.

Rabe, E. vd. (2003). "Bonner Venenstudie der Deutschen Gesellschaft für Phlebologie" *Phlebologie* 32: 1– 14.

Raj, T. vd. (2008). "Intestinal microbial contribution to metabolic leucine input in adult men" J Nutr. 2008; 138(11): 2217–21.

Raju, S., Fredericks, R., Lischman, P., Neglen, P., Morano, J. (1993). "Observations on the calf venous pump mechanism: determinants of postexercise pressure" *J Vasc Surg.* 17: 459–469

Rapprich, S., Dingler, A., Podda, M. (2011). "Liposuction is an effective treatment for lipedema-results of a study with 25 patients" J Dtsch Dermatol Ges. 9(1):33–40

Rapprich, S., Baum, S., Kaak, I., Kottmann, T., Podda, M. (2015). "Treatment of lipoedema using liposuction: Results of our own surveys" *Phlebologie.* 44: 121–132.

Rawlings, A.V. (2006). "Cellulite and its treatment" *Int J Cosmet Sci.* Jun;28(3):175-90. doi: 10.1111/j.1467-2494.2006.00318.x.

Redolfi, S., Arnulf, I., Pottier, M., Bradley, T.D., Similowski, T. (2011). "Nocturnal rostral fluid shift: a unifying concept for the pathogenesis of obstructive and central sleep apnea in men with heart failure" Respir Physiol Neurobiol. Mar 15; 175(3): 390-393.

Reich-Schupke, S., Gahr, M., Altmeyer, P., Stücker, M. (2009). "Resting pressure exerted by round knitted moderate-compression stockings on the lower leg in clinical practice – results of an experimental study" *Dermatol Surg* 35: 1989–1997

Reich-Schupke, S., vd. (2014). "Efficacy and comfort of medical compression stockings with low and moderate pressure six weeks after vein surgery" *Phlebology* 29: 358– 66.

Reich-Schupke, S., Murmann, F., Altmeyer, P., Stücker, M. (2009). "Quality of life and patients' view of compression therapy" 28: 385– 93

Reich-Schupke, S., Altmeyer, P., Stücker, M. (2012). "Pilotstudie zur Kompressionsversorgung von Patienten mit Lipödem, Lymphödem und Lipolymphödem" *LymphForsch* 16: 65–69

Reich-Schupke, S., Mohren, E., Stücker, M. (2018). "Survey on the diagnostics and therapy of patients with lymphedema and lipedema" *Hautarzt* 69: 471–477

Reich-Schupke, S., Stücker, M. (2019). "Round-knit or flat-knit compression garments for maintenance therapy of lymphedema of the leg? - Review of the literature and technical data" *J Dtsch Dermatol Ges.* Aug;17(8): 775-784. doi: 10.1111/ddg.13895.

Reich-Schupke, S., Stücker, M. (2018). "Individualisierte Kompressionstherapie" *Der niedergelassene Arzt* 09: 75–76

Rebuffe-Scrive M. vd. (1985). "Fat cell metabolism in different regions in women. Effect of menstrual cycle, pregnancy, and lactation" *J. Clin. Invest.* 75, 1973–1976

Ris, H.B., Furrer, M., Stronsky, S., Walpoth, B., Nachbur, B. (1993). "Four-compartment fasciotomy and venous calf-pump function: long-term results" *Surgery* 113: 55–58

Robinson, E. vd. (2013). "Eating attentively: a systematic review and meta-analysis of the effect of food intake memory and awareness on eating" *Am J Clin Nutr.* 97(4):728-742.

Robson, A.A. (2013). "Preventing the Epidemic of Non-Communicable Diseases: An Overview". Bioactive Food as Dietary Interventions for Liver and Gastrointestinal Disease. Edited by R.R. Watson, V.R. Preedy, Chapter 25, 383-400.

Rocha, L.A., Ferreira de Almeida, E.B.L., Gontijo Filho, P.P. (2009). "Changes in hands microbiota associated with skin damage because of hand hygiene procedures on the health care workers" *Am J Infect Control* 37: 155–159.

Rocher, M. vd. (2020). "Benefits of Outdoor Sports in Blue Spaces. The Case of School Nautical Activities in Viana do Castelo" Int J Environ. Res. Public Health. 17(22): 8470.

Rockson, S.G. (2009). "The unique biology of lymphatic edema" *Lymphat Res Biol.* 7: 97–100.

Romani, A.M. (2011). "Cellular magnesium homeostasis" Arch. Biochem. Biophys. 512: 1–23.

Rook, G.A.W., Martinelli, R., Brunet, L.R. (2003). "Innate immune responses to mycobacteria and the downregulation of atopic responses" *Current Opinion in Allergy and Clinical Immunology.* 3 (5): 337–342.

Ropacka-Lesiak, M., Kasperczak, J., Breborowicz, G.H. (2012). "Risk factors for the development of venous insufficiency of the lower limbs during pregnancy—part 1" *Ginekol Pol.* 83(12): 939–942

Rushmer, R.F. (1970). "Effects of posture" *Cardiovascular dynamics. 3rd ed.* WB Saunders, Philadelphia; 192–219

Ryan TJ. (1995). "Lymphatics and adipose tissue". Clinics in Dermatology 13.5: 493-498.

Ryu, K. H. , Shin, H. S. , Yang, E. Y. (2015). "Effects of laughter therapy on immune responses in postpartum women" *Journal of Alternative and Complementary Medicine*, 21(12), 781–788. 10.1089/acm.2015.0053

Sachdev, H.S. vd. (2005). "Anthropometric indicators of body composition in young adults: relation to size at birth and serial measurements of body mass index in childhood in the New Delhi birth cohort" *Am J Clin Nutr* 82: 256–266

Sadick, N.S. (1992). "Predisposing factors of varicose and telangiectatic leg veins" J Dermatol Surg Oncol 18: 883-886.

Saint-Auban, E. (1929). "La Chirurgie Esthe´tique" *Revue des grands proce`s contemporains: recueil d'e´loquence judiciaire,* Paris. Ed. Emile de Saint-Auban, 191–227, 226.

Sajantila, A. (2013). "Major historical dietary changes are reflected in the dental microbiome of ancient skeletons" Investig Genet 4: 10.

Sakula, A. (1984). "In search of Hippocrates: a visit to Kos" J R Soc Med 77: 682–688

Sarosiek, J., Scheurich, C.J., Marcinkiewicz, M., McCallum, R.W. (1996). "Enhancement of salivary esophagoprotection: rationale for a physiological approach to gastroesophageal reflux disease" *Gastroenterology* 110(3): 675-681

Sarwer, D.B., Wadden, T.A., Pertschuk, M.J., Whitaker, L.A. (1998). "Body image dissatisfaction and body dysmorphic disorder in 100 cosmetic surgery patients" Plastic & Reconstructive Surgery, 101, 1644-1649.

Sasaki, S., Katagiri, A., Tsuji, T., Shimoda T., Amano K. (2003). "Self-reported rate of eating correlates with body mass index in 18-y-old Japanese women" *Int. J. Obes.* 27(11):1405–1410

Schemann, M., Neunlist, M. (2004). "The human enteric nervous system" Neurogastroenterol Motil 16 (Suppl 1): 55–59

Schmeller, W., Meier-Vollrath, I. (2007). "Lipödem-aktuelles zu einem weitgehend unbekannter Krankheitsbild" *Aktuelle Dermatologie* 33:1–10

Schmeller, W., Hueppe, M., Meier-Vollrath, I. (2012). "Tumescent liposuction in lipoedema yields good long-term results" Br J Dermatol. 166(1): 161–168

Schneider, M., Conway, E.M., Carmeliet, P. (2005). "Lymph makes you fat" *Nature Genetics,* vol. 37, no. 10, 1023-1024

Schnepper, R., Richard, A., Wilhelm, F.H., Blechert, J. (2019). "A combined mindfulness-prolonged chewing intervention reduces body weight, food craving, and emotional eating" *J Consult Clin Psychol.* 87(1):106-111.

Schroeder, H.A. (1971). "Losses of vitamins and trace minerals resulting from processing and preservation of foods" *Am J Clin Nutr.* 24: 562–573

Schwartz, S.I., Brunicardi, F.C. (2010). "Schwartz's Principles of Surgery" 9. New York: McGraw-Hill, Medical Pub. Division

Scully, J.L. (2004). "What is a disease?" *EMBO Rep.* Jul; 5(7): 650–653, doi: 10.1038/sj.embor.7400195

Sebastian, A., Frassetto, L.A., Sellmeyer, D.E., Morris, R.C. Jr. (2006). "The evolution-informed optimal dietary potassium intake of human beings greatly exceeds current and recommended intakes" Semin Nephrol. Nov; 26(6): 447-53.

Selhub, J., Jacques, P.E., Wilson, P.W. vd. (1993). "Vitamin status and intake as primary determinants of homocysteinaemia in an elderly population" JAMA 270: 2693-2698.

Seligman, M.E.P., Csikszentmihalyi, M. (2000). "Positive psychology: an introduction" *Am. Psychol.* 55 5–14

Sellayah, D., Cagampang, F.R., Cox, R.D. (2014). "On the Evolutionary Origins of Obesity: A New Hypothesis" Endocrinology, Volume 155, Issue 5: 1573–1588,

Shadid, S., Jensen, M.D. (2003). "Effects of pioglitazone vs diet and exercise on metabolic health and fat distribution in upper body obesity" Diabetes Care 26: 3148–3152

Sharma, S.P., Chung, H.J., Kim, H.J., Hong, S.T. (2016). "Paradoxical Effects of Fruit on Obesity" *Nutrients* 8(10):633. Published 2016 Oct 14. doi:10.3390/nu8100633

Shaw, B.H., Claydon, V.E. (2014). "The relationship between orthostatic hypotension and falling in older adults" Clin. Auton. Res. 24, 3–13

Sheikhrohani, S. (2003). "Investigating relationship of identity status with anxiety and age, gender and education level" Thesis of MA, Ferdowsi Mashad University.

Siervo, M., Wells, J.C., Cizza, G. (2009). "The contribution of psychosocial stress to the obesity epidemic: An evolutionary approach" *Horm Metab Res.* 41: 261–70.

Sihota, J., Shannon, S., Bhattacharyya, A. (2007). "History taking" *Learning to consult.* Charlton Rodger (ed.) Radcliffe Publishing; 10–28

Silver, T. (1990). A New Face on the Countryside: Indians, Colonists, and Slaves in South Atlantic Forests, 1500-1800. New York,Cambridge University Press, 35-9

Silvestris, E., de Pergola, G., Rosania, R., Loverro, G. (2018). "Obesity as disruptor of the female fertility" Reprod Biol Endocrinol. Mar 9; 16(1): 22

Simeon, D., Grantham-McGregor, S. (1987). "Cognitive function, undernutrition, and missed breakfast" *Lancet.* 2: 737–738

Simmons, A.H. (2011). *The Neolithic Revolution in the Near East: Transforming the Human Landscape,* Tucson, AZ: University of Arizona Press

Smith, G.D., Greenwood, R., Gunnell, D. vd. (2001). "Leg length, insulin resistance, and coronary heart disease risk: The Caerphilly Study" J Epidemiol Community Health 55: 867–872. 10.1136/jech.55.12.867

Snell, B., Fullmer, S., Eggett, D.L. (2014). "Reading and listening to music increase resting energy expenditure during an indirect calorimetry test" *J Acad Nutr Diet.* 114(12): 1939-1942.

Snijder M. B. vd. (2004). "Trunk fat and leg fat have independent and opposite associations with fasting and postload glucose levels: the Hoorn study" *Diabetes Care* 27, 372–377

Snijder, M. B. vd. (2004). "Independent and opposite associations of waist and hip circumferences with diabetes, hypertension and dyslipidemia: the AusDiab Study" *Int. J. Obes. Relat. Metab. Disord.* 28, 402–409

Soest, T., Kvalem, I.L., Roald, H.E., & Skolleborg, K.C. (2009). "The effects of cosmetic surgery on body image, self-esteem, and psychological problems" Journal of Plastic, Reconstructive & Aesthetic surgery, 62(10), 669-679.

Somers, P., Knaapen, M. (2006). "The histopathology of varicose vein disease" *Angiology* 57(5): 546–555

Speakman, J.R. (2016)i "Evolution of Obesity. In: Ahima R.S. (eds) Metabolic Syndrome" *Springer, Cham Evolution of Obesity* 103-122

Stallworth, J.M., Hennigar, G.R., Jonsson, H.T. Jr, Rodriguez, O. (1974). "The chronically swollen painful extremity. A detailed study for possible etiological factors" *JAMA* 228: 1656–1659

Stanhope, J.M. (1975). "Varicose veins in a population of lowland New Guinea" Int J Epidemiol. 4: 221-225.

Stearns, S. (1998). *Evolution in Health and Disease* Oxford: Oxford University Press

Stern, S.E. vd. (2005). "Identification of individuals with insulin resistance using routine clinical measurements" Diabetes. 54(2): 333–339.

Stevens, D.L. vd. (2014). "Practice guidelines for the diagnosis and management of skin and soft tissue infections: 2014 update by the Infectious Diseases Society of America" Clin Infect Dis 59(2): e10-52.

Stewart, J.M., Karman, C., Montgomery, L.D., McLeod, K.J. (2005). "Plantar vibration improves leg fluid flow in perimenopausal women" m J Physiol Regul Integr Comp Physiol. Mar; 288(3): R623-9.

Stiemsma, L.T., Nakamura, R.E., Nguyen, J.G., Michels, K.B. (2020). "Does Consumption of Fermented Foods Modify the Human Gut Microbiota?" J Nutr. Jul 1;150(7): 1680-1692. doi: 10.1093/jn/nxaa077. PMID: 32232406; PMCID: PMC7330458.

Stranden, E., Kroese, A.J. (1998). "Venodynamics in healthy subjects and in patients with venous dysfunction" *Scope on Phlebology and Lymphology* 5: 4–12.

Strauss, A., Hubbe, M., Neves, W.A., Bernardo, D.V., Atuí, J.P. (2015). "The cranial morphology of the Botocudo Indians, Brazil" Am J Phys Anthropol. Jun; 157(2): 202-16.

Strohmeier, K. vd. (2022). "Multi-Level Analysis of Adipose Tissue Reveals the Relevance of Perivascular Subpopulations and an Increased Endothelial Permeability in Early-Stage Lipedema" Biomedicines, May 18; 10(5): 1163 doi: 10.3390/biomedicines10051163.

Ströhle, A., Hahn, A., Sebastian, A. (2010). "Estimation of the diet-dependent net acid load in 229 worldwide historically studied hunter-gatherer societies" American Journal of Clinical Nutrition. 91(2): 406–412.

Struckmann, J.R. (1987). "Assessment of venous muscle pump function by ambulatory calf volume strain gauge plethysmography after surgical treatment of varicose veins: a prospective study of 21 patients" *Surgery* 101: 347–353

Stutz, J.J. (2011). "Liposuction in lipedema to prevent later joint complications" *Vasomed* 23:6

Succurro, E. vd. (2008). "Insulin secretion in metabolically obese, but normal weight, and in metabolically healthy but obese individuals" *Obesity (Silver Spring)* 16(8): 1881–1886

Suga, H. vd. (2009). "Adipose tissue remodeling in lipedema: adipocyte death and concurrent regeneration" *Journal of Cutaneous Pathology,* vol. 36, no. 12, 1293–1298

Sun, K., Tordjman, J., Clément, K., Scherer, P.E. (2013). "Fibrosis and adipose tissue dysfunction" *Cell Metabolism,* vol. 18, no. 4, 470–477

Sundman, E., Olofsson, P.S. (2014). "Neural control of the immune system" Adv Physiol Educ 38:135–139

Swartz, M.N. (2004). "Clinical practice. Cellulitis" N Engl J Med. 350:904–912.

Szabo, A., Ainsworth, S.E., Danks, P.K. (2005). "Experimental comparison of the psychological benefits of aerobic exercise, humor, and music" *Humor* 18: 235-246

Szél, E., Kemény, L., Groma, G. vd. (2014). "Pathophysiological dilemmas of lipedema" *Med Hypotheses.* 83(5): 599–606.

Szolnoky, G., Kemény, L. (2010). "Lipoedema: from clinical presentation to therapy Further aspects" *Br J Dermatol.* 162(4):889. doi: 10.1111/j.1365-2133.2009.09619.x.

Szolnoky, G., Nemes, A., Gavaller, H., Forster, T., Kemeny, L. (2012). "Lipedema is associated with increased aortic stiffness" Lymphology 45:71-79.

Tanaka, T. vd. (2008). "Tsujimoto G. Free fatty acids induce cholecystokinin secretion through GPR120" Naunyn Schmiedebergs Arch Pharmacol 377:523–527

Taubes, G. (2013). "The science of obesity: what do we really know about what makes us fat?" *BMJ* 346:f1050. 10.1136/bmj.f1050

Tchernof, A., Despres, J.P. (2013). "Pathophysiology of human visceral obesity: an update" Physiol Rev. 93(1): 359–404.

Teimourian, B. (1997). "Ultrasound-assisted liposuction" *Plast Reconstr Surg* 100:1623–1625.

Teixeira, P.J. vd. (2010). "Mediators of weight loss and weight loss maintenance in middle aged women" *Obesity (Silver Spring)* 18:725–735

Tekiner, H. (2018). "Hastalık yok, hasta vardır: Hermann Hesse'nin Çarklar Arasında Romanı Üzerine Tıbbi Değerlendirmeler (There is no disease but the patient: Medical observations on Hermann Hesse's Novel Beneath the Wheel)" *Türkiye Biyoetik Dergisi,* Vol. 5, No. 4, 198-199

Terranova, F., Berardesca, E., Maibach, H. (2006) "Cellulite: nature and aetiopathogenesis" *Int J Cosmetic Science* 28: 157–167

The Journal of Christopher Columbus (During His First Voyage), and Documents Relating to the Voyages of John Cabot and Gaspar Corte Real, Clements R. Markham, ed. and trans. (London: 1893), 37-68.

Thomae, H.J. (2013). “Grundlagen” *Moderne Kompressionstherapie,* S. Reich-Schupke, M. Stücker. Köln, Viavital, 13– 32.

Thursby, E., Juge, N. (2017). “Introduction to the human gut microbiota” Biochem. J. 474:1823–1836.

Tidhar, D., Katz-Leurer, M. (2009). “Aqua lymphatic therapy in women who suffer from breast cancer treatment-related lymphedema: a randomized controlled study” *Support Care Cancer.* 18:383–392

Tiedjen, K.U., Schultz-Ehrenburg, U., Holzmann, H., Altmeyer, P., Hör, G. (1985). “Isotopenlymphographische Befunde beim Lipödem“ *Dermatologie und Nuklearmedizin.* Berlin: Springer-Verlag; 432-438

Tiedjen, K.V., Knorz, S. (1992). “Different methods of diagnostic imaging in lymphedema, lipedema and venous disorders: indirect lymphography, xeroradiography, CT and isotope lymphography” *Progress in lymphology: XIII, International Congress of Lymphology* Amsterdam: Elsevier Science Publishers B.V. 521-524

Tinetti, M.E., Williams, C.S., Gill, T.M. (2000). “Dizziness among older adults: A possible geriatric syndrome” Ann. Intern. Med. 132, 337–344

Tinkle, B., vd. (2017). “Hypermobile Ehlers-Danlos syndrome (a.k.a. Ehlers-Danlos syndrome Type III and Ehlers-Danlos syndrome hypermobility type): clinical description and natural history” *Am J Med Genet C Semin Med Genet.* 175:48–69

Tooby, J., Cosmides, L. (1990). “The past explains the present: emotional adaptations and the structure of ancestral environments” *Ethol. Sociobiol.* 11, 375–424. doi: 10.1016/0162-3095(90)90017-Z

Tooby, J., Cosmides, L. (1992). “The psychological foundations of culture” *The Adapted Mind: Evolutionary Psychology and the Generation of Culture,* ed. J. Barkow, L. Cosmides, and J. Tooby, New York, NY: Oxford University Press

Torre, Y.S., Wadeea, R., Rosas, V., Herbst, K.L. (2018). “Lipedema: friend and foe” Horm Mol Biol Clin Investig 33. doi:10.1515/hmbci-2017-0076

Trevathan, W.R., McKenna, J.J., Smith, E.O. (eds) (1999). *Evolutionary Medicine*, Oxford University Press, New York

Trott, S.A. vd. (1999). “Sensory changes after traditional and ultrasound-assisted liposuction using computer-assisted analysis” *Plast Reconstr Surg* 103:2016–2025; discussion: 2026-2028

Tudoraşcu, I. vd. (2014). “Motor unit changes in normal aging: A brief review” *Rom J Morphol Embryol.* 55:1295–1301

Turnbaugh, P.J. vd. (2007). “The human microbiome project” Nature 449: 804–810.

Turnbaugh, P.J. vd. (2009). “A core gut microbiome in obese and lean twins” *Nature* 457: 480–484.

Tsatsoulis, A., Mantzaris, M.D., Bellou, S., Andrikoula, M. (2013). “Insulin resistance: an adaptive mechanism becomes maladaptive in the current environment - an evolutionary perspective” Metabolism. May; 62(5): 622-33.

Uhl, J.F., Gillot, C. (2010). « The plantar venous pump: Anatomy and physiological hypotheses” Phlebology 16:12 Page 151

Xu, Y., Lopez, M. (2018). “Central regulation of energy metabolism by estrogens” Mol Metab 15:104-115.

Van Dam, N.T. vd. (2018). “Mind the Hype: A Critical Evaluation and Prescriptive Agenda for Research on Mindfulness and Meditation” Perspect Psychol Sci. Jan; 13(1): 36-61.

Van de Pas, C.B. vd. (2020). “Does tumescent liposuction damage the lymph vessels in lipoedema patients?” Phlebology, 35(4):231-236. doi: 10.1177/0268355519885217. Epub

2019 Nov 1.

Van der Velden, S.K., Shadid, N.H., Nelemans, P.J., Sommer, A. (2014). "How specific are venous symptoms for diagnosis of chronic venous disease?" *Phlebology* 29:580–586. doi: 10.1177/0268355513515859

Van der Wegen-Franken, C.P., Mulder, P., Tank, B., Neumann, H.A. (2008). "Variation in the dynamic stiffness index of different types of medical elastic compression stockings" *Phlebology* 23: 77– 84.

Van der Wegen-Franken, C.P., Tank, B., Nijsten, T., Neumann, H.A. (2009). "Changes in the pressure and the dynamic stiffness index of medical elastic compression stockings after having been worn for eight hours: a pilot study" *Phlebology* 24: 31–37

Van Dijk, N., Wieling, W. (2009). "Fainting, emancipation and the 'weak and sensitive' sex" J Physiol. 587 (Pt 13): 3063-3064

Van Geest, A.J., Esten, S.C.A.M., Cambier, J-P.R.A. vd. (2003). "Lymphatic disturbances in lipedema" *Phlebologie*. 32:138–142

"Varicose veins in the legs: the diagnosis and management of varicose veins" (2013). National Institute for Health and Care Excellence; London (UK) Available: www.nice.org.uk/guidance/index.jsp?action=byID&o=14226 (accessed 2013 July 31)

Varilla, C., Marcone, M., Paiva, L., Baptista, J. (2021). "Bromelain, a Group of Pineapple Proteolytic Complex Enzymes *(Ananas comosus)* and Their Possible Therapeutic and Clinical Effects. A Summary" Foods. Sep 23; 10(10): 2249.

Vazquez, G., Duval, S., Jacobs, D.R., Silventoinen, K. (2007). "Comparison of body mass index, waist circumference, and waist/hip ratio in predicting incident diabetes: a meta-analysis" Epidemiol Rev. 29: 115–128.

Vieth, R. (2020). "The Paleolithic Nutrition Model in Relation to Ultraviolet Light and Vitamin D" In: Reichrath, J. (eds) Sunlight, Vitamin D and Skin Cancer. Advances in Experimental Medicine and Biology, vol 1268.

Vitaterna, M.H., Takahashi, J.S., Turek, F.W. (2001). "Overview of circadian rhythms" Alcohol Res Health. 25(2): 85-93.

Vitellaro-Zuccarello, L., Cappelletti, S., Dal Pozzo Rossi V., Sari-Gorla, M. (1994). "Stereological analysis of collagen and elastic fibers in the normal human dermis: variability with age, sex, and body region". *The Anatomical Record.* 238 (2): 153–162.

Vrdoljak, J. vd. (2022). "Effects of Olive Oil and Its Components on Intestinal Inflammation and Inflammatory Bowel Disease" Nutrients. Feb 11;14(4): 757. doi: 10.3390/nu14040757. PMID: 35215407; PMCID: PMC8875923.

Vormann, J. (2016). "Magnesium: Nutrition and Homoeostasis" AIMS Public Health. May 23; 3(2): 329-340.

Vos, E. (2000). "Whole grains and coronary heart disease" *Am J Clin Nutr* 71: 1009

Wahls, T.L., Chenard, C.A., Snetselaar, L.G. (2019). "Review of Two Popular Eating Plans within the Multiple Sclerosis Community: Low Saturated Fat and Modified Paleolithic" Nutrients. Feb 07; 11(2)

Walter, J., Ley, R. (2011). "The Human Gut Microbiome: Ecology and Recent Evolutionary Changes" *Annual Review of Microbiology* 65: 1, 411-429

Wang, H.D., Zheng, J.H., Deng, C.L. vd. (2008). "Fat embolism syndromes following liposuction" Aesthetic Plast Surg. 32: 731–736

Wannamethee, S.G., Shaper, A.G., Whincup, P.H. (2005). "Alcohol and adiposity: effects of quantity and type of drink and time relation with meals" Int J Obes 29: 1436–1444

Warren Peled, A., Kappos, E.A. (2016). "Lipedema: diagnostic and management challenges" *Int J Womens Health* 8:389-395

Watve, M.G., Yajnik, C.S. (2007). "Evolutionary origins of insulin resistance: a behavioral switch hypothesis" BMC Evol Biol. Apr 17; 7:61

Waxler, J.L. vd. (2017). "Altered body composition, lipedema, and decreased bone density in individuals with Williams syndrome: a preliminary report" Eur J Med Genet 60:250-256.

Weddell, J.M. (1969). "Varicose veins pilot survey" Br J Prev Soc Med 23: 179-186.

Weiss, E.C., Galuska, D.A., Kettel Khan, L., Gillespie, C., Serdula, M.K. (2007). "Weight regain in U.S. adults who experienced substantial weight loss, 1999–2002" *Am J Prev Med* 33: 34–40

Welch, G.N., Loscalzo, J. (1998). "Homocysteine and atherothrombosis" N Eng J Med 338: 1042-1050.

Wells, J.C.K. (2012). "Obesity as malnutrition: the role of capitalism in the obesity global epidemic" American Journal of Human Biology. 24: 261–276.

Wells, J.H., Hurvitz, K.A. (2011). "An evidence-based approach to liposuction" *Plast Reconstr Surg.* 127:949.

Wengle, H.P. (1986). "The psychology of cosmetic surgery: Old problems in patient selection seen in a new way—Part 2" *Ann Plast Surg.* 16: 487

Widmer, L.K. (1978). "Peripheral venous disorders: prevalence and socio-medical importance: observations in 4529 apparently healthy persons", Basle Study III, Berne, Switzerland, Huber.

Wilson, G.T. (1994). "Behavioral treatment of obesity: thirty years and counting" *Adv. Behav. Res. Ther.* 16:31–75. doi: 10.1016/0146-6402(94)90002-7

Wiedman, D. (2012). "Native American Embodiment of the Chronicities of Modernity: Reservation Food, Diabetes, and the Metabolic Syndrome among the Kiowa, Comanche, and Apache" Medical Anthropology Quarterly. 26:599–600.

Willard, C. (2019). "6 Ways to Practice Mindful Eating: Informal mindfulness practices for those of us who don't have five minutes to contemplate a raisin" Avaible: https://www.mindful.org/6-ways-practice-mindful-eating/

Williams, G.C. (1957). "Pleiotropy, natural selection, and the evolution of senescence" *Evolution* 11: 398-411

Williams, G.W., Nesse, R.M. (1991). "The dawn of Darwinian medicine" *Q Rev Biol* 66: 1-22

Wokaunn, M., Ferenčić, S.F., Mikolaučić, M. (2013). "The pictogram of the pes planus from the first century AD" *Int Orthop.* 37(9):1871-1873. doi:10.1007/s00264-013-2020-4

Wold, L.E., Hines, E.A. Jr, Allen, E.V. (1951). "Lipedema of the legs; a syndrome characterized by fat legs and edema" Ann Intern Med 34:1243-1250.

Wollina, U. (2017). "Lipedema: up-to-date of a long forgotten disease" https://www.ncbi.nlm.nih.gov/pubmed/28493139 *Wien Med Wochenschr.* 67: 343–348

Wollina, U., Heinig, B. (2019). "Treatment of lipedema by low-volume micro-cannular liposuction in tumescent anesthesia: Results in 111 patients" Dermatol Ther. 32(2):e12820

Woo, P.C., Lum, P.N., Wong, S.S., Cheng, V.C., Yuen, K.Y. (2000). "Cellulitis Complicating Lymphoedema" Eur J Clin Microbiol Infect Dis. 19:294–297.

Wrangham, R., Conklin-Brittain, N. (2003). "Cooking as a biological trait" Comp Biochem Physiol A Mol Integr Physiol. Sep; 136(1): 35-46

Yamada, S. (2011). "Walking just after a meal seems to be more effective for weight loss than waiting for one hour to walk after a meal" *Int J Gen Med.* 4:447-450. doi:10.2147/IJGM.S18837

Yoshikawa, Y. vd. (2019). "Beneficial effect of laughter therapy on physiological and psychological function in elders" *Nurs Open.* Jan; 6(1): 93–99.

Yudkin, J. (1978). "Dietary factors in arteriosclerosis: sucrose" *Lipids* 13: 370–372

Yumino, D. vd. (2010). Nocturnal rostral fluid shift: a unifying concept for the pathogenesis of obstructive and central sleep apnea in men with heart failure. Circulation. Apr 13; 121(14):1598-605.

Zandian, M., Ioakimidis, I., Bergh, C., Brodin, U., Södersten, P. (2009). "Decelerated and linear eaters: effect of eating rate on food intake and satiety" *Physiol Behav* 96:270–275

Zhang, R.Z., Gashev, A.A., Zawieja, D.C., Davis, M.J. (2007). "Length-tension relationships of small arteries, veins, and lymphatics from the rat mesenteric microcirculation" Am J Physiol 292: H1943–1952

Zhang, X., Adamson, R.H., Curry, F.E., Weinbaum, S. (2008). "Transient regulation of transport by pericytes in venular microvessels via trapped microdomains" PNAS 105: 1374–1379

Zak, P.J. (2015). "Why inspiring stories make us react: the neuroscience of narrative" Cerebrum. Feb 2; 2.

Zawieja, D. (2005). "Lymphatic biology and the microcirculation: past, present and future" *Microcirculation*. 12: 141–50

Zeisel, S.H., Mar, M.H., Howe, J.C., Holden, J.M. (2003). "Concentrations of choline-containing compounds and betaine in common foods" *J Nutr.* 133: 1302–1307

Zweifach, B.W., Prather, J.W. (1975). "Micromanipulation of pressure in terminal lymphatics in the mesentery" Am J Physiol 228: 1326–1335

Made in United States
Orlando, FL
04 November 2026

90200814R00125